Praise fo

"The exploration into one's own personal sexuality that Mali and Joe encourage is like a key that opens the door to our truest nature. Most of all, this book is about intimacy—not the quick fix, but the real, deep, authentic intimate connection that everyone is searching for. The kind of intimacy that's truly sustainable."

~Isabel Mize, Marriage and Family Therapist

"This will definitely be my go-to book for clients who are in long-term 'couplings' and are interested in understanding, enhancing, and deepening the connection in their relationships—in and out of the bedroom."

~Dr. R. Y. Langham, Marriage and Family Therapist & Family Psychologist

"Mali Apple and Joe Dunn have once again created literary magic with this deeply engaging book on love, life and relationship. Wonderful and inspiring!"

~Paul Samuel Dolman, Host of the *What Matters Most* Podcast

"If you have ever wondered if a monogamous relationship will inevitably become boring, stale and stagnant, then this book will blow your mind! Mali and Joe have captured the sizzling secrets to bring spice, fun and spontaneity into every relationship and to make monogamy the hottest choice around. Curl up with this book and then cuddle up with your partner and prepare for the most sensual, spicy and sexy relationship you could ever imagine—without ever changing partners!"

~Michelle Marchant Johnson, Dating Coach with Love Life Coaching

Wild Monogamy

Also by Mali Apple & Joe Dunn

The Soulmate Experience: A Practical Guide to Creating Extraordinary Relationships

The Soulmate Lover: A Guide to Passionate and Lasting Love, Sex, and Intimacy

Free Resources

Get your free bonus materials for *Wild Monogamy* at www.MaliAndJoe.com/WildMonogamyResources

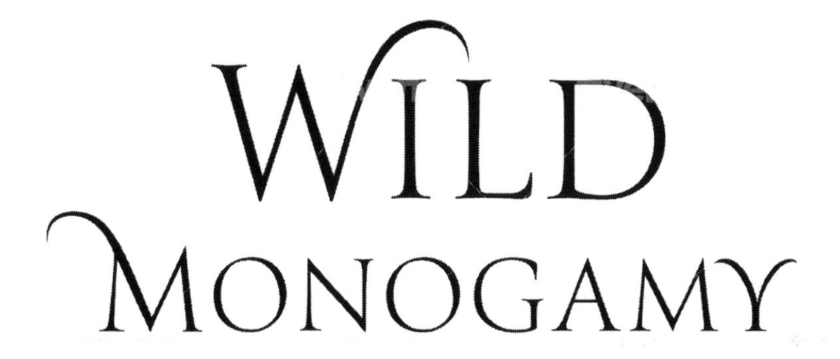

Wild Monogamy

Cultivating Erotic Intimacy to Keep Passion and Desire Alive

MALI APPLE & JOE DUNN

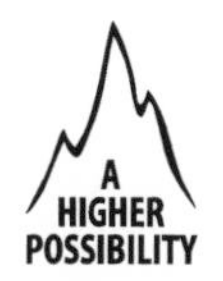

San Rafael, California

Published in the United States by A Higher Possibility, San Rafael, California.
www.ahigherpossibility.com

Editor: Yolanda D'Aquino

Cover design: Robin Locke Monda

Publishers Cataloging-in-Publication Data

Names: Apple, Mali, author. | Dunn, Joseph, 1958--, author.

Title: Wild monogamy : cultivating erotic intimacy to keep passion and desire alive / Mali Apple and Joe Dunn.

Description: Includes bibliographical references and index. | San Rafael, CA: A Higher Possibility, 2023.

Identifiers: LCCN: 2022916682 | ISBN: 978-0-9845622-8-2 (print) | 979-8-9869262-0-9 (ebook) | 979-8-9869262-1-6 (audio)

Subjects: LCSH Love. | Sex. | Intimacy (Psychology). | Interpersonal relations. | BISAC FAMILY & RELATIONSHIPS / Marriage & Long-Term Relationships | FAMILY & RELATIONSHIPS / Love & Romance | HEALTH & FITNESS / Sexuality | FAMILY & RELATIONSHIPS / Dating

Classification: LCC HQ23 .A68 2023 | DDC 306.7--dc23

ISBN 978-0-9845622-8-2

First Edition

www.MaliAndJoe.com

Notes to Readers

All personal stories in this work are true. Names have been changed, identifying details have been altered, and some stories have been combined out of respect for the privacy of individuals and couples.

This book is not a substitute for counseling, therapy, or medical treatment, and the advice and strategies it contains may not be suitable for every situation. This book is sold with the understanding that the publisher and authors are not engaged in rendering medical, legal, or other professional services, and the authors and publisher assume no responsibility for any loss, damage, or malady caused by the information or lack of information it contains. Please consult with trained professionals about any matters that may require diagnosis or medical attention.

The fact that an individual, organization, or website is cited in this work or mentioned as a potential source of further information does not mean that the authors or publisher endorse the information that individual, organization, or website provides or recommendations they may make.

To the many extraordinary people who allowed us
to share their stories in these pages. You will touch the
lives and hearts of so many others.

And to our team of angels, who kept us inspired
and on task. We are forever grateful for your
unwavering belief in us.

CONTENTS

INTRODUCTION

For their fifteenth anniversary, Kyle and Lauren left their sons with a family friend and went away for a long weekend. They had spent months anticipating the trip and were looking forward to finally spending some time alone.

Kyle and Lauren love each other and are happy with the life they've created together. But because their primary focus over the past decade had been on building their careers and raising their family, their own relationship had unintentionally become less of a priority.

"We were very excited to have the chance to reconnect as a couple—and reclaim our chemistry!" said Lauren.

"We took along a couple of sexy games we'd bought for the occasion," Kyle told us. "We made ourselves wait until we'd checked into our room and were stretched out on the bed before we opened them. An hour later, we were both feeling completely depressed!"

Lauren said they found the suggestions for role-play scenarios and sex positions boring and predictable.

"I was utterly uninspired," she said.

"We were looking at each other like, 'Is this all there is?'" Kyle said.

"What about passion?" Lauren asked. "How do we tap into that deeper, sexy feeling of connection?"

Answering that question is exactly what motivated us to write *Wild Monogamy*.

A risqué game, a creative technique, or a new sex toy might be just what some couples are looking for. But for Lauren and Kyle, a new location and some ideas for novelty and fun just weren't enough. What they were really seeking were ways to reconnect with that exciting feeling of possibility and aliveness they knew was within reach. Like so many couples, they wanted to develop—or redevelop—what we call erotic intimacy.

Drawing on current research in the fields of relationships and sexuality, as well as on the experiences of everyday people from all walks of life, *Wild Monogamy* is a diverse collection of ways for couples to develop and deepen their erotic connection and intimacy. You'll discover how to

- initiate provocative conversations about love, intimacy, and sex—and keep them going
- enhance your emotional intimacy and build resilient trust
- keep your sexual connection a priority while juggling work, family, and other responsibilities
- support each other in exploring the edges of your erotic comfort zones
- apply the healing power of eroticism to help free each other from fears, anxieties, insecurities, shame, and self-consciousness
- approach common intimacy issues as opportunities for self-awareness, pleasure, and growth
- not only transcend jealousy, but transform it into passion
- design your own intimate adventures
- continually fire up your mutual attraction and desire—as well as your mutual pleasure!

Through their inspiring personal accounts, people we've interviewed and coached reveal an abundance of creative ways they've applied these concepts. These courageous individuals share stories of how they have approached a range of issues affecting their sexual and emotional bond, as well as how they've explored their desires and discovered new levels of connection with their partners. You'll witness the incredible intimacy that's generated when two people help each other expand their erotic comfort zones or find a new way to work with a sexual fear, challenge, or inhibition.

Since our own anecdotes are often of value to others, we're willing to be vulnerable and share our (blushingly personal!) stories with you, too. This is a good place to mention that we're not trained therapists or health care professionals. If we were, it's unlikely we would be so candid. We're just two people who are fascinated by the question of how to keep a long-term relationship compelling, connected, sexy, and fun—a question we've been exploring, and answering, since we met two decades ago.

Now, no single book has all the answers, which is one reason we've listed some of our favorite relationship and sexuality books in the Resources section. In addition, if you have a medical issue that's impacting you sexually, it's important to seek proper care. If you are being affected by previous trauma or abuse, we highly recommend working with a counselor or therapist. And if you have very little or no sexual connection, or raising the topic makes your partner defensive or angry, other issues in your relationship might need addressing. Consulting a professional can help you understand and address those concerns.

If you have a good relationship but your partner isn't interested in reading this book themselves, that's okay. You'll no doubt find a suggestion for a conversation or exploration that intrigues them or a sexy new twist on something you two already enjoy. You'll also likely gain new perspectives on any issues you've been having, which can help you find more positive and effective approaches to those challenges.

Finally, we know that some percentage of couples will, at some point, consider having an intimate experience with another person or persons. For these couples, the last chapter explores how to have honest and loving conversations about this possibility as well as how to compassionately work with any fears, insecurities, or jealousies so that the experiences are positive and rewarding for everyone involved.

So let's jump right in! The sooner we do, the sooner you can discover how to create a more dynamic, more exciting relationship that has a solid foundation of love and trust and becomes even more intimate as time goes on. It's precisely that solid foundation that will make it possible to continually cultivate erotic intimacy—and keep your passion, desire, and pleasure fully alive.

1

CIRCLES AND EDGES

Once you become a couple, it's typical to begin drawing an imaginary circle around yourselves. This "relationship circle" is formed by your beliefs, ideas, and assumptions about relationships—often acquired from and shaped by family and friends, the media, previous relationships, and society in general. These beliefs and ideas have a great influence on how you approach your roles and your responsibilities and what you expect from each other and from the relationship. Your circle is also defined by any agreements or rules you make together, such as how you will or won't behave with certain people or in certain situations. Your intention in creating this circle is to protect the love and happiness the two of you have found together.

For some couples, the circle they create works quite well and reflects their shared values and visions for the relationship. But for others, all those beliefs, agreements, and expectations can have unintended consequences. Issues can arise when partners assume their ideas about relationships are more or less identical, when in reality they might differ substantially. For example, two people might both say—and believe—that monogamy is important to them, but their specific ideas about what being monogamous means may vary in significant ways. Couples' contradictory assumptions about what is and isn't included in their circle have been the cause of endless disagreements, confusion, and heartache.

When couples draw their relationship circle too tightly around themselves, they leave little or no space for mystery or curiosity. Even couples who are generally happy with the circle they've created together might find that the romance, emotional intimacy, or sexual vitality between them eventually begins to subside. When this happens, their relationship can feel less compelling. Without knowing how to prevent this decline, they may one day resign themselves to the idea that this is simply what happens in a long-term relationship.

Biologically speaking, growth and change are key elements of what it means to be alive. So for a relationship to feel alive, it must grow and evolve. Change doesn't have to be constant or extreme. Just a bit now and then will help keep the excitement level a little higher all the time.

If you're in a relationship, you can invite growth and change—and make space for a little mystery—by first getting a clear sense of the relationship circle the two of you have created. And if you're single, it will be tremendously valuable to understand what could influence any future circle you might take part in creating. So let's get started.

WHAT DEFINES YOUR CIRCLE?

For a moment, imagine how your relationship might look if you created your relationship circle intentionally instead of letting your unexamined beliefs or conditioning define it for you. Would it be more harmonious? More exciting? More fun? Less work?

To consciously create your relationship circle, you have to start by assessing what's currently defining your circle or what has defined any you have had in the past. The questions in the Intimacy Inquiry that follows are designed to illuminate your beliefs and values around romantic relationships in general and monogamy in particular. There are three primary ways to use this inquiry: contemplating the questions on your own, exploring them with your partner, or using them as intimate conversation starters with someone you're dating.

Reflecting on these questions on your own will give you insight into yourself and how you've approached relationships in the past. When you become aware of what has been unconscious in your attitudes and behaviors, you can start to implement positive changes that will make your relationship much more satisfying.

If you and your partner are willing to come together and take a fresh look at what you've created together, talking about even just a few of these topics can profoundly strengthen your connection. For one, the vulnerability required to share your feelings on topics like these in itself builds understanding and trust and deepens intimacy. Even if you've been together for decades, you'll find these conversations both educational and stimulating. They may offer you new insights into any challenges you are facing together. And they will likely lead to other interesting conversations—and even explorations—of your own.

Unless both of you are ready to dive into all of the questions, choose just those that you're both open to exploring. If you don't feel ready for a particular topic, take the time to look at why not. If you're comfortable talking about the reasons for your reluctance, that alone can be an excellent opportunity for more understanding and connection between you.

There's no right or wrong here. You're just sharing some of the ideas and beliefs you each hold. And there's no need to rush the process. You might just take a question or two along with you on a walk or out to dinner.

Some couples really enjoy the deep conversations these questions inspire. Other couples, such as those dealing with unresolved trust or anger issues, might be unable to comfortably talk about any of these topics. If this describes your situation, imagine for a moment what it would be like if you *could* talk about them. How would that feel? What would make such conversations possible? Reflecting on these questions can start to shift the way you relate to each other in subtle but positive ways.

If you're single, the Intimacy Inquiry will give you an understanding of how your attitudes, beliefs, values, and upbringing have influenced your prior relationships—and might influence them in the future.

The topics in the Intimacy Inquiry are also well worth exploring with a new or prospective partner. The intimate conversations these questions inspire will help you get to know each other better and discover whether your values, attitudes, and desires are compatible. Sharing your beliefs and ideas on these topics from the start, and listening to each other with receptivity, sets the tone for an open, honest approach to your relationship while building genuine trust. By consciously constructing your circle in this way, the two of you will be actively designing your most rewarding—and exciting!—relationship possible.

THE INTIMACY INQUIRY

How you feel about the questions that follow will be influenced by a number of factors, including your social or spiritual upbringing, your past relationships and sexual experiences, and the degree of intimacy you feel in your current relationship. Although many of these are phrased as yes-or-no questions, your responses will likely be much more layered and complex. Your feelings on any particular topic might vary according to context and may have evolved over time, all of which makes for richer discussions.

As you read through the questions in each category, notice any reactions or emotions that surface. These responses provide useful information. For instance, if a question makes you uncomfortable and you can't identify why, the topic may be worth deeper investigation and is an opportunity to learn something important about yourself or your partner.

Also keep in mind that these questions are just a discovery process and starting points for mind-expanding and heart-opening conversation. Use them in whatever ways suit you best.

Romantic Love

- What does it mean to you to be in love?
- Is there a difference between loving someone and being in love with them?
- What does "I love you" mean to you?
- Have your ideas about romantic love changed over time?

Intimacy

- What does intimacy mean to you?
- How does intimacy make you feel?
- How important is intimacy to you?
- What does "being intimate" mean to you?
- Is there a difference between having sex and making love?

Emotions

- Do you believe that some emotions are positive or good while others are negative or bad? For example, is anger bad? Is sadness undesirable?
- Are there acceptable and unacceptable ways of expressing emotions?
- How comfortable are you with your own emotions?
- How comfortable are you with your partner's emotions?

Personal Space and Time

- How much space or time to yourself do you need in a relationship? How much space and time do you want to share with your partner?
- When you're socializing or attending an event together, how important is it to you to spend time by each other's side? How important is it to you to mingle independently?
- Is it desirable or undesirable to have separate goals, plans, or interests? Do you feel that independent pursuits will reduce or enhance your intimacy? Why?

Monogamy

- Do you believe that monogamy is the best way to have a successful relationship, the only way, or just one way?
- What do you appreciate about monogamy?
- What do you find challenging or frustrating about monogamy?

Sex in a Monogamous Relationship

- Do you think it's inevitable that a couple's sexual connection will taper off over time? Or do you believe it's possible to keep a monogamous relationship sexually interesting and exciting over many years?

Agreements

- What are some agreements you think are generally accepted between couples and don't need discussing? What about agreements that are generally accepted between couples but could actually benefit from some discussion?
- Did you have any agreements in prior relationships that didn't work for you? Did you ever face a challenging situation involving an unspoken agreement in a previous relationship?
- Have you and your partner established any agreements about what is okay and not okay when it comes to sex in general or your sexual relationship in particular?

- Can you think of any unspoken agreements or assumptions between you?
- How would you want to handle it if one of you broke an agreement the two of you have?

Your Pasts

- Do you believe that one's previous relationships and sexual experiences should be kept private from one's current partner?
- Do you think there are times when sharing stories about your romantic pasts, previous lovers, or sexual histories can be positive or important? If so, under what circumstances, and how much detail would you be comfortable with?

Relationships with Former Partners

- How do you feel about maintaining friendships with previous partners, assuming they are good people in general and the relationship wasn't toxic or traumatizing?
- Is it okay to text or call an ex to wish them happy birthday? What about getting together to catch up on each other's lives?
- Are you interested in getting to know your lover's former partners if possible? Or would you prefer that mentions of them be avoided or reminders of them be kept out of sight?

Friendships

- Do you feel it's inappropriate for you or your partner to have close friends of a certain gender, relationship status, or level of attractiveness? Or do you believe that such friendships can bring benefits to your relationship? If so, how?
- Have you ever said or felt that it's inappropriate for your partner to pursue a particular friendship? Have you ever tried or wanted to restrict your partner from spending time with someone?

Affection with Others

- Is being physically affectionate with people other than your partner or immediate family members okay—holding hands, walking arm in arm, sharing a long hug, greeting with a kiss? Would your feelings depend on who they were or whether or not you were there?

Conversations About Sex

- Is sex a common, comfortable, or even exciting topic of conversation in your relationship? Or are conversations about sex awkward, filled with conflict, infrequent, or even nonexistent?
- Is it okay for you or your partner to talk with friends about sex? How about discussing your sex life in particular?

Nudity

- Are you comfortable being naked—by yourself, with your partner, in the presence of other people?
- How do you feel about public nudity, such as at nude beaches, clothing-optional resorts, skinny-dipping sites, or events like Burning Man or Mardi Gras?
- How comfortable would you be if your partner were naked in any of these environments, with or without you there?

Media and Privacy

- What value do you place on each other's privacy?
- Do you ever monitor each other's online activity or discourage each other from showing interest in certain websites, videos, or articles?
- How do you feel about having access to each other's phone, email, or social media accounts?
- Do you believe that you or your partner developing friendships through the internet is okay or a cause for concern?

Sexual Fantasies

- What are your feelings about someone in a committed relationship fantasizing about other people?
- Should you both feel free to engage and enjoy your sexual imaginations in whatever ways you choose, or do you think certain types of fantasies are harmful and should be off limits?

- Is there a place for fantasy in a loving relationship?
- Are you open to hearing your partner's fantasies, sharing your own, or pursuing some of your fantasies together?

Erotica

- What types of erotic materials—books, magazines, movies, online stories, photos, or videos—are acceptable or unacceptable for one or both of you to consume? When, what, and how much is okay or not okay?
- Do you feel that any erotica or pornography at all will detract from your relationship in some way or is even a form of cheating? Or are you comfortable with such material within certain guidelines—for example, as long as it involves consenting adults, isn't watched when the kids are awake, or isn't negatively affecting your relationship?
- Would you be open to reading or watching some kinds of erotica together, perhaps as a way to share your interests or as a source of new ideas?

Attraction to Others

- Do you think your partner should be sexually attracted to no one other than you?
- How do you feel about either of you going without the other to dance clubs, strip clubs, or bachelor or bachelorette parties?
- When you're out together, do you feel you should both make an effort not to take too much notice of others, or is looking at other attractive people with appreciation okay? How much looking is acceptable and what would be too much?
- Are you comfortable telling your partner when you notice someone attractive? Are you comfortable with your partner telling you when they notice someone attractive?
- Are you comfortable telling your partner when you're feeling uneasy about their attention toward someone else?

Public Displays of Affection

- Are you relaxed holding hands, hugging, or kissing in public, or do you avoid most public displays of affection?
- Are there circumstances where some displays of affection in public would feel more or less comfortable to you?

Flirting

- Do you believe that people in committed relationships should never flirt with someone else? Or do you think flirting with others can be beneficial for a relationship? If so, why, and what kinds of flirting would you be comfortable with?
- Do you tell your partner when you think someone is attracted to you? When you think someone is attracted to them? When you're feeling an attraction to someone else? Or do you keep observations like these to yourself?

Sexual Activities

- How sexually adventurous have you been in the past? How sexually adventurous are you now?
- How adventurous do you think your partner is?
- Are there any relatively common sexual activities—such as dirty talk, oral sex, masturbation, anal sex, or light bondage—that you particularly enjoy? Are there any that make you feel uncomfortable?
- Do you have a desire or willingness to explore sexuality together? Do either of you have an interest in trying new things? Is this an interest you share? What would you be interested in trying and what seems like it might be too far out of your comfort zone?
- How might you feel if your partner seemed uncomfortable about a sexual activity you have an interest in?
- And finally, what do you love most about sex—both in general and with your partner?

People will come to these questions from many different perspectives, circumstances, and experiences. Some people will feel very at ease with this entire self-assessment. For others, contemplating these questions may bring up challenging emotions or highlight difficulties that they have been grappling with.

If you're having a hard time with some or possibly many of these questions, and especially with the thought of talking about them with your partner, that's okay. As you consider the information and ideas in this book, your comfort level will gradually increase and it will feel easier and more natural to begin having conversations about some of these topics.

If reading through and discussing all of these questions was easy for you and you feel there's not much growth for you to experience in any of these categories, we have one more question for you to think about: *What is one area where you personally could make a small shift that would have a positive effect on the intimacy in your relationship?*

If you're single, still take time to reflect on your beliefs around each of these topics. Then, when you're starting a new relationship, remember to return to the Intimacy Inquiry—both to gain perspective on your new connection and for some potent conversation starters. Having interactions like these from the start will help you consciously create an environment of authentic intimacy—giving your new relationship true erotic potential!

EXPANDING YOUR EROTIC EDGES

There are as many ways to have a passionate, compelling, and satisfying relationship as there are people to have them. Because every couple is different and every relationship is unique, the secret is to design your *own* relationship style, one that works best for the two of you. The conversations inspired by the Intimacy Inquiry will help you and your partner determine what will keep your unique relationship, and your sexual connection, feeling fresh and alive.

Because you've had different childhoods, different experiences, and different influences, it's almost inevitable that your belief systems—and thus your relationship circles—won't line up perfectly. By getting a good sense of what defines your circle and what defines your partner's circle, you'll be able to see where your values and beliefs align. This area of alignment defines your shared relationship circle and is where you feel most comfortable together.

The smaller your shared circle, the sooner your sex life may start to feel routine and predictable. When you try to feel content within a small, inflexible circle, never trying anything that would make either of you uneasy, sooner or later you might find yourselves feeling bored. Even if there's variety in your sexual repertoire, if you never expand to include anything new, or even just talk about the possibility of something new, you still might experience the fading of passion and desire over time.

There are, of course, many couples who are genuinely happy and content with a relationship that is largely unchanging. But a substantial percentage of couples eventually grow dissatisfied with the predictable and uninspiring sex that can characterize a long-lasting relationship. Happily, the best things about being in a committed relationship—the familiarity, the sense of safety and belonging, the mutual love and support—are also what can make your shared circle a solid foundation for inviting in a little mystery and adventure.

So here's a proposition. Start thinking of what's just outside the edges of your shared circle as *future possibilities*. Whether it's an edge for you, an edge for your partner, or an edge for both of you, slowly expanding these "erotic edges" together can be all it takes to continually fire up your desire for each other and keep your sexual connection energized.

In the chapters that follow, we'll be sharing stories from real couples, along with an abundance of creative ideas, to give you plenty of inspiration for expanding your erotic edges. Along the way, you'll be oh-so-gently encouraged to cultivate a "yes" attitude toward sexual exploration and to continually evolve your idea of what sex is and can be.

One way to expand an erotic edge is by exploring something that has you both feeling a little nervous or shy. Sex can be so many (wonderful!) things: an endlessly erotic and sensual physical activity, an infinitely creative endeavor, a loving expression of emotional connection, a profoundly transformational or even mystical experience. As a couple, no matter your ages or how long you've been together—and even if you've experienced difficulties with arousal, erections, or orgasms—being willing to explore in all these realms gives you unlimited sexual potential together. And the erotic intimacy that you'll be developing will lead to experiences that are so pleasurable and meaningful—and for some, even spiritual—that you'll remember them among the peak moments of your life.

A second way to expand an erotic edge is to experiment with something that's an edge for just one of you, while the other offers loving encouragement and guidance into the new territory. Rather than being a possible source of misunderstanding or frustration, the differences between your circles become phenomenal opportunities for intimacy—and fun!

You've probably already discovered that sex has a way of bringing to the surface unacknowledged or unhealed issues in us. Almost all of us have suffered from feelings of insecurity, anxiety, guilt, or embarrassment around some aspect of sexuality. The stories in this book of the many loving and creative ways that couples have acknowledged, explored, and transformed such feelings will move and inspire you. You'll see how difficulties involving body image, self-esteem, shame, physical limitations, sexual inhibitions, and performance anxiety can be extraordinary opportunities for intimacy, healing, and growth. Supporting each other in becoming free of whatever is keeping you from experiencing love and pleasure will be some of the most gratifying and memorable experiences the two of you will ever share.

As you continue to expand your erotic edges, you'll be developing a foundation of trust, acceptance, and love. Your shared circle will become a circle of safety, connection, and sexy anticipation—an erotic sanctuary in which you can dream up your next adventure, and your next, and your next. All of which will make the yeses come much more easily!

2

SIX KEYS TO INTIMATE ADVENTURES

For most of us, to keep our relationship and our sexual connection exciting, every once in a while we have to explore something new. We have to have some sort of intimate adventure.

An intimate adventure is simply anything that feels exciting to the two of you. There are endless possibilities, like spending a sexy evening planning an erotic weekend getaway—or reminiscing about your last one! Adventures don't have to be happening all the time. You just need to feel that the potential for them exists. A little sparkle and excitement every so often is enough to keep a relationship charged with sexual energy all year round.

Before you explore the many kinds of intimate adventures presented in this book, we encourage you to become familiar with the six keys in this chapter:

- connection
- communication
- trust
- acceptance
- mutual support
- gratitude

These six keys are the foundation for creating an environment that ensures not only that your explorations keep your sex life exciting, but that you grow more connected through them. That's because trying something new can involve supporting each other in developing more self-confidence, for example, or letting go of a doubt or fear, or healing from something that happened in the past. Whether your adventures are purely physical, deeply emotional, or focused on creativity and fun, these six keys are essential to making them a success.

CONNECTION COMES FIRST

In any intimate adventure, connection comes first—and for good reason. Being fully connected with each other around whatever you're planning means you'll be enjoying those feelings of anticipation and excitement *together*. Attempting something new or edgy when you're *not* feeling connected, on the other hand, can do more harm than good by triggering feelings of doubt, fear, or mistrust.

To create experiences that feel positive and passionate to you both, it's imperative that you don't move forward unless you're moving forward *together* and that you stay connected at every step along the way. From sharing your fears and desires, to conjuring up future erotic possibilities, to supporting each other through the process, make your connection a priority in every aspect of your sexual relationship.

When one of you proposes something new—like experimenting with a creative idea or playing out a certain fantasy—remember that it can take courage and vulnerability to even make such a suggestion. This is true even when you've known someone a long time (perhaps *especially* when you've known someone a long time!). Remembering this will help to create a receptive space in which the two of you can talk openly about a new possibility, including what excites you about it, what makes you nervous, and what it might be like to actually make this possibility a reality.

It's also vital that you both come to any adventure with a true desire for it. Make it perfectly okay for either of you to say, "I'm not sure," "not just yet," or "that's just not for me" to any proposal without being judged for it. Often people will say yes because they're embarrassed to share their real feelings or afraid they'll be spoiling the fun. Or they might feel pushed into something they're not yet ready for or interested in. Be sure every yes—yours and your partner's—is an authentic yes. Reluctance is most definitely not the feeling you want to be taking into a sexual adventure!

If your partner expresses curiosity about a particular activity and you're not sure if what you're feeling in response is a yes or a no, be honest about your ambivalence while keeping an open mind. Say something like, "I'm intrigued. Not ready to say yes yet, but intrigued. Let's keep talking!"

When your go-to response to new ideas is receptivity and you make connection your priority, just exploring a new proposal together can be incredibly exciting—no matter how far you eventually take it or whether you ever actually try it at all. We've been tossing around some crazy ideas for years that we may never go all the way with, and that's just fine. Because of our connection, it's a turn-on just to ponder possibilities. And it has led to a lot of spontaneous fun!

With connection as your intention, you'll be more in tune with your partner and have a better sense of what small step might be just enough of a stretch. For instance, suppose Melissa would like to visit the adult store downtown, but her husband Eric is apprehensive. By talking about whatever it is that makes Eric nervous, they might find ways to alleviate his concerns. If he's afraid he'll feel intimidated, for example, they could visit the store's website to get more comfortable with what they might find if they visited in person. If he's worried that the people there will be too weird or creepy (or that they'll think Melissa and Eric are weird and creepy!), they can make a pact to leave at any moment if one of them wants to, without resistance, complaint, or annoyance from the other. Such an agreement makes it safer and easier for a couple to enter unfamiliar territory together, as they both know they can change their yes to a no at any time.

Or suppose Eric would like to experiment with some bondage in the bedroom, but the prospect makes Melissa a little uneasy. One small step they might take in that direction is to look together at some videos or books on the subject. If part of the issue is that Melissa doesn't see anything sexy or sensual about either restraining someone or being restrained, they could—if she's willing—read or listen to some erotic stories that involve light bondage. If she's interested, they could then start with something very simple, like a blindfold, and Eric could do everything in his power to *make* the experience sensual and connecting for her, like whispering in her ear, "What if I just hold your hands together while I kiss your neck the way you love so much?"

In both of these situations, it's essential to recognize that Eric and Melissa's connection is their first priority, not the satisfaction of one or the other's desire. Focusing on their shared connection creates a feeling of safety and togetherness and allows them to explore these new arenas in ways that are exciting for them both.

Whether it's visiting a shop that sells sex toys, trying out a little bondage, or anything else that makes one or both of you nervous, the more you've talked about the possibilities beforehand, the more connected you will feel if you decide to move in that direction. Ask each other questions that draw out your feelings:

- What makes you nervous about this? What excites you about it?
- How would you want us to respond if this or that happens?
- How can we ensure that we're both enjoying ourselves all the way through this experience?

If and when you choose to take that next step, stay true to your intention to maintain your connection the entire time. Let's say you've decided to attend an erotically themed festival or costume party. Before you enter that environment, take a moment to check in and remind yourselves that you're here to have fun together while staying completely connected. With this as your focus, you'll be there to support each other if needed, addressing any fears or apprehensions that come up or taking a break to reconnect if things start feeling awkward or overwhelming. When your connection is truly your priority, "Let's stop, I've had enough" really means "Let's stop, *we've* had enough"!

After any intimate adventure, give yourselves plenty of opportunity to talk about anything that surfaced during the encounter or that you found yourself reflecting on later—observations, insights, realizations, or something that surprised you. Talking about the erotic escapades you've had is one of the most exciting and connecting things about having them—not to mention giving you plenty of inspiration for your *next* adventure!

It's sexy and satisfying to create such depth of connection with another human being. In fact, you might find that beyond just being the priority during your erotic explorations, your connection eventually becomes the very purpose of pursuing them. Your connection—which makes everything you do together more fulfilling, exciting, and fun—becomes its own reward.

THE OTHER ORAL SEX

When I (Mali) was entering puberty, I began secretly raiding the "dirty books" my dad had stashed under the old pajamas and mismatched socks in his bottom dresser drawer: *The Happy Hooker, The Sensuous Man, The Sensuous Woman, The Story of O.* Although all the descriptions of sexual activities and techniques fascinated me, I was especially captivated by the story of a woman and her visiting lover having "oral sex" on her living room couch. This potent phrase, my curious mind reasoned, must certainly mean "talking about sex." And was I ever intrigued! I fantasized for hours on end about the day when my future (handsome and sexy) boyfriend and I would cuddle on the couch and engage in long, steamy sessions of "oral sex."

Just as communication is universally recognized as one of the keys to a successful long-term relationship, an open and ongoing dialogue around your sex life and your sexual interests can elevate your emotional intimacy. Besides, talking about sex is arousing! Indulging in some verbal foreplay over a romantic dinner is one of the sexiest things you can do with your clothes on. Conversely, if you *can't* talk about sex—your dreams and your desires, your fantasies and your fears, or some tantalizing new idea—your sex life probably isn't as stimulating or satisfying as it could be.

Whether it's reminiscing about an encounter you had together, bringing up some kinky sex practice you've read about, or sharing a story from your past, "oral sex" keeps you turned on. Infusing your everyday interactions with sexy banter can fuel your desire for each other indefinitely.

Couples with full lives and family obligations may find that "oral sex" is sometimes the only sex they have time for. If these are your current circumstances, keep the dialogue open by acknowledging that: "We both know how challenging this is right now. We have to remember that one day we'll have more time for long lovemaking sessions. In the meantime, let's do what we can to keep our sexual connection alive." Then make sure to have a quick sexy exchange as often as you can. Whisper in your partner's ear what you'd like to do to them the next time you're alone together. Leave them a little love note or send a flirtatious text ("You're so hot—I can't wait until you get home!"). If one of you is out of town for work, set aside twenty minutes for some good old-fashioned phone sex. By keeping the conversation about sex going, you keep sex within easy reach (or at least easier reach!).

Open, honest, and ongoing communication is also a must for making any kind of sexual exploration successful. There's an idea, perpetuated by movies and porn, that once you start making love, you stop making conversation. Yet being able to communicate during sex—such as asking, "How is this for you, sweetie? What can I do to make it even better?"—can lead to more connection and more fun. A new experience can provoke unexpected feelings of uncertainty, insecurity, fear, or jealousy in either of you, so being able to express and explore your reactions is essential. Becoming comfortable talking about sex will also make it easier to move through any sexual issues or problems that might arise.

Many people, however, are more comfortable having sex than talking about it. So how do you get more comfortable talking about sex? It's simple. If you intentionally make sex a regular topic of conversation, you'll become more relaxed about it.

Yes, there will probably be moments of awkwardness, but that's a *good* thing. Feeling uncomfortable and vulnerable is part of what makes intimacy, well . . . intimate! Even a conversation about why a particular topic makes one or both of you nervous or unsure can be very connecting. It will also give you valuable insight—not only into your partner, but also into yourself.

If you're both up for exploring a provocative question, you might try one of these:

- What sensual memory comes to mind from when you were young?
- Tell me about your first good kiss.
- Do you remember any sexual dreams you've had?
- What sexual experiences have we had together that stand out to you or that you'd like to try again?

- How might our sex life be different if we felt totally free and uninhibited?

If you're thinking that your partner would never be up for conversations like these, we'd like to suggest you keep an open mind. Unless they're adamantly shutting you down (in which case, seeking out some counseling is probably a good idea), try bringing up a spicy subject or two once in a while. Just keep the topics simple and the tone light. Even more importantly, don't pressure your partner to be interested or even to respond, and remind yourself in advance not to have any expectations. I (Mali) have enticed more than a few men I was dating into sexy conversations. It just took an attitude of invitation and an intention to make it safe and fun for them to join in.

Also remember that your different childhoods, personalities, sexual histories, and life experiences will influence how comfortable you each feel with any particular topic. Some things will be easy for one or both of you to talk about, while others might be challenging. One person may find it fun (or exciting) to tell the story of when and where they learned about various aspects of sex. The other, perhaps because of painful experiences they've had or just being more shy or reserved, might need a lot of time and positive interactions together before they feel safe enough to open up about something so personal (if they ever do). Partners can also have very different comfort levels with hearing the other talk about certain topics.

There are unlimited sources of sexy conversation starters. Read up on sexual techniques, such as erotic massage, fellatio, or cunnilingus. Pick up a classic like the Kama Sutra or *The New Joy of Sex*, or something more current and cutting edge. Subscribe to informative sex and relationship podcasts or start following experts in the fields of eroticism and relationships on social media. Also, be sure to check out the advanced "oral sex" questions in chapter 7. You can even plan a date night where all non-tantalizing topics are off-limits: no work talk, no politics, no complaints. Instead, spend dinner conversing about the sensual aspects of the meal, arousing recollections you have, a risqué experience you've been planning, or what you're going to do to each other later that evening.

Conversations about sex can, of course, be highly charged. They have the potential to stir up fears and insecurities, troubling memories, or feelings of embarrassment and shame. If you and your partner have had unsettling or angry interactions about sex in the past, you're probably not ready for these types of conversations, let alone intimate adventures that push your boundaries. In that case, consider working with a professional who can facilitate conversations about sexuality and help you dive beneath the surface of your emotional reactions and understand where those responses are coming from. This way, you'll be able to improve your communication skills and learn to be more open to each other's perspectives.

Becoming more comfortable talking about sex, and learning to listen to each other with openness and receptivity, will vastly increase the chances that your shared sexual explorations will be enjoyable and positive. By talking well in advance about something you might want to try one day, you'll both know when you're feeling ready to go ahead. These conversations will keep the sexual energy alive between you, even if you never make that particular prospect happen. In fact, there are times when the delicious electricity you spark by verbally exploring all the details and nuances of a proposal can feel even more erotic than the experience itself.

On a summer trip to Las Vegas, we spent a few hours at a well-known sex club on the outskirts of town—and the titillating conversations leading up to our visit were every bit as exciting as walking through the door. We went with no intention of engaging with anyone else; we were in Vegas, we knew that having adventures together keeps things exciting, and the club was there! Stepping inside was like stepping back in time: the beaded curtains and strings of pom-poms, the velvet couches, the vintage porn playing on the big screen. The most interesting interaction we had there was our conversation with the parking lot attendant. He'd been working at the club for thirty years and had seen it all! We felt like a couple of undercover private investigators. We did manage to sneak off to an empty room, so at least we can say we've had sex at a sex club. And the fun didn't end when, our mission complete, we made our way back to our hotel. We imagine we'll be talking about that escapade for a long time to come!

Now I (Joe), unlike Mali, did not grow up fantasizing about cuddling up with my girlfriend on the couch and talking about sex. But I'm happy to step into the role of Mali's fantasy man, as I can attest that these conversations keep us erotically charged up. Not only do we have a blast, but talking about sex also results in having more sex. And I'm all for that!

RESILIENT TRUST

When asked to name the most important elements of a successful relationship, people often put trust near the top of their list. Unfortunately, in many relationships trust is built upon fairly shaky foundations. What is commonly referred to as trust often involves unspoken expectations about what one's partner will and won't do, in the sense of "I trust you to do this—and I trust you *not* to do that!" But this kind of trust can't offer a relationship a solid support.

Trust isn't something that can be imposed, on either a partner or a relationship. Real trust is cultivated over time, through qualities like these:

- **Communication.** Pay attention to how you communicate. For example, avoid using accusations or put-downs, and apologize if you slip up. When your partner is speaking, give them your full attention rather than mentally rehearsing what you're going to say next.

- **Awareness.** When a conflict arises, honestly assess your own beliefs and motivations, and make an effort to see the situation from both perspectives. And remember to take your partner into account when you're making decisions that affect them.
- **Reliability.** Follow through on what you say you will do, and resist the urge to make promises you're not sure you can keep. If you're running late, let your partner know with a call or text. Own up to your actions—and your inactions—rather than putting the blame somewhere else.
- **Trustworthiness.** Be someone your partner can count on when they need advice, assistance, or a shoulder to cry on. Keep any confidences or secrets they share with you strictly private. And finally, be honest. Show your partner that whatever you say can be believed, even when the truth might be hard to hear.

These guidelines may seem obvious, but you still might find them challenging to follow all the time. Fortunately, life will give you plenty of opportunities to practice!

Like most things in a relationship, it takes two to build trust. The presence or absence of the qualities we've listed above can be a good indication of whether or not a partner, or prospective partner, is worthy of your trust.

Before we continue, it's important to say that if there's a history of dishonesty or deception between you, we encourage you to give your relationship careful examination. Either find a skilled counselor to help you work through that distrust or, if that's not possible, consider whether you need to leave the relationship.

There is a certain degree of trust that two people can develop if they agree never to do anything beyond their comfort zones and both stay true to that agreement over time. Sex therapist David Schnarch calls this "untested trust."[1] This is a healthy level of trust that can serve a couple's relationship perfectly and indefinitely—as long as they never stretch the limits of their comfort zones. Because their trust hasn't been tested, however, they don't know how strong or reliable it actually is.

Trust that *has* been stretched and expanded a little at a time, and strengthened through that process, is what we call *resilient trust*.

You and your partner can cultivate resilient trust by supporting each other in expanding your comfort zones—including your erotic edges—together. Such experiences create a deeper sense of safety and stability in your relationship. With resilient trust, you'll be far better prepared to venture into uncharted territory together. You'll be ready to handle the unexpected, such as an emotional reaction either of you might have that couldn't have been anticipated. Eventually you will simply both *know* that you will find your way back to a connected place whenever you experience a disconnection. Resilient trust is trust you can rely on.

Building resilient trust is a gradual process. So whatever new idea or adventure you're considering, don't take a giant leap. Start with something small, simple, and manageable. You both want to feel excited, and even a little nervous, but not insecure or freaked out. Let's say that Austin has a desire to try some kind of anal play, but Jackie is apprehensive. They could first try incorporating some small aspect of that activity into their sex life, such as some light touching or massaging of that area, without moving beyond what Jackie feels ready for. If Jackie's need for safety and comfort is honored and Austin's desire to eventually take things further is guided by true concern for Jackie's wellbeing, the trust between them will continue to build. Jackie may slowly become more relaxed with their explorations and willing to experiment a little more.

Over time, as you both develop ways to work through whatever reactions new experiences tend to bring up for you, you'll come to trust that you both will always try to do what you feel is best for the two of you and the relationship. As you build resilient trust, you'll be inspired to venture a little further out on your edges—because you will know that whatever comes up, you'll be able to find your way through it together and grow stronger and more connected in the process.

AN ATTITUDE OF ACCEPTANCE

When we're able to be our authentic selves with each other, we can reveal what's really going on for us. In order to share ourselves this honestly and openly, we need to know we're in a safe, supportive, and nonjudgmental environment. A vital component of creating such an environment is acceptance.

Acceptance allows us the freedom to be ourselves in each other's presence. It is acceptance that makes real intimacy possible.

As with most things in a relationship, acceptance starts with yourself. Whether it's quieting your self-criticism, healing from shame or guilt, or growing more comfortable in your body and with your sexuality, self-acceptance is a lifelong process.

Many people struggle to accept certain aspects of their own sexuality. The fear of being considered strange or rejected for our sexual interests, fantasies, or experiences—or, perhaps even worse, having actually been ridiculed or rejected for them in the past—is very common. This almost universal fear is not without good reason. We've been conditioned to think that any sexual interest outside the narrow range of what most people consider "normal" is weird, deviant, or perverted, so we may judge ourselves harshly for an interest or fantasy that is, in reality, perfectly normal and healthy.

The truth is, practically everyone has their own set of turn-ons: ideas, images, scenarios, or activities that intrigue or excite them. When approached in a thoughtful and responsible way, the vast array of sexual interests that humans can have reveal exciting and novel ways for a couple to explore together. For this reason, sexual individuality—including our different sexual interests, fantasies, histories, and experiences—is something we should be celebrating rather than fearing.

Your partner's sexual interests, like yours, probably have been with them for a long time and were not consciously chosen.[2] Accepting that your partner has a particular fantasy or desire doesn't mean you have to take it on for yourself. That said, their interest is unlikely to go away any time soon, and if it isn't illegal, harmful, or something you know for sure you'll never feel comfortable with, it can be of great benefit to your relationship to at least try to develop an understanding of it. You might even be able to find a variation of it that you *can* participate in. If you're willing to consider exploring it with them, even in a small way, you'll find yourself with a very appreciative partner.

Developing an attitude of acceptance toward sexual desires and proclivities requires thoughtfulness, especially because people often equate acceptance with approval. What's essential to understand is that *acceptance doesn't mean agreement or approval.* It doesn't mean you have to participate in someone else's interest or that they have to participate in yours. Acceptance is simply acknowledgment. Being receptive, open-minded, and nonjudgmental toward yourself and others means that you acknowledge whatever thoughts, feelings, and desires are present. It means not shaming or ridiculing yourself or your partner and having compassion for any guilt or shame that exists around a particular interest. It also helps to understand that, in most cases, we don't choose our sexual interests—it's more like they choose us. Unless they're causing difficulty or leading to harmful behaviors, almost all sexual desires and fantasies are perfectly normal and okay. And although our fantasies and desires may evolve as we age, changing the things that excite us can be very challenging and is often just not possible.[3]

Unconditional acceptance is the foundation of an ever-deepening emotional bond. When you know that there is mutual acceptance between you, it's much easier to relax, let down your guard, and reveal more of who you are. In that protective space, erotic intimacy can truly flourish.

BE THERE NOW

To grow closer and more connected through your intimate adventures, you need to be able to count on one another for support, guidance, and encouragement. You need to *be there now* for each other.

You may be familiar with the concept of "be here now," popularized by spiritualist Ram Dass's 1971 book of the same name, about being present in the moment. "Be there now" speaks to being present *for your partner* in the moment. Having a shared intention to be there for each other is essential for building resilient trust and will ensure that your adventures are fulfilling for both of you. This foundation of mutual support will make you stronger as a couple, and you'll become more and more devoted to each other over time.

We all have our challenges around sexuality: fears, jealousies, insecurities, physical limitations, areas of shame or regret. Whether it's self-consciousness about some aspect of our bodies or how they function, a habit of comparing ourselves to others and feeling deficient, a fear of being touched in a particular way or seen in a certain position, or embarrassment about our desires and interests, things can and will arise for us when we're expanding our sexual comfort zones.

For someone who's experienced trauma or abuse or who suffers from a debilitating anxiety, there might be too many current challenges to be psychologically or emotionally ready for new sexual adventures that stretch their boundaries. Part of being there for your partner is making sure that every yes they give to a suggestion or activity is an enthusiastic, full-body yes. Also be aware if your partner's enthusiasm seems to diminish or you notice a shift in them, such as a feeling of disconnection or the sense that something is going unsaid. Expressing your willingness to be there for them at that moment can be healing in and of itself and will often restore the connection between you.

When you're experimenting with new things sexually, know that the reality can turn out to be quite different from the vision or the fantasy. You and your lover might talk for hours about an idea, delving into exactly what about the scenario intrigues each of you, any nervousness or hesitation you feel, and how you plan to stay connected throughout the experience. You might both feel you're ready to move forward, that you have a good sense of how things will go—and the reality of the situation can still surprise you. You can never know for sure what's going to happen when you try that new activity or walk through that next door together. Sometimes the experience might not be as enjoyable as you anticipated, for one or both of you. Or the partner whose idea it was might find themselves disappointed, while the other, who originally may have had some doubts, might get right into it.

Also, be aware that no matter how comfortable you feel going in, unusual experiences can stir up unexpected insecurities, jealousies, or memories of a bad or traumatic experience—even some you thought you had worked through long ago. Out of a sense of embarrassment, a desire to appear more confident than you actually feel, or not wanting to adversely affect what's happening, you might be inclined to ignore, deny, or hide such things. Yet when both of you are committed to being there for each other, sharing these moments is a unique opportunity for connection and growth.

Here's a great example of this. Claudia, a college professor, attended an intimacy workshop with her girlfriend. At some point during one of the exercises, a feeling of panic swept over her.

"I wasn't sure what to do," Claudia recalls. "For a few moments I tried to cover it up, but it was overwhelming. When I confessed to Kaye that I was feeling really scared, she put her arms around me and held me. At that moment, I felt closer to her than I ever had before."

Before any new experience, know that fears, anxieties, and insecurities might come up for either of you, and commit in advance to supporting each other in whatever ways are needed. This requires a relationship environment that allows you both to express feelings of discomfort or uncertainty at any time. You each need to be able to say, "You know, I thought I'd enjoy this, but I'm feeling a little strange and I don't even know why." Being there for each other could mean shifting your attention to that feeling for the time being: "Let's slow down and talk about what's happening for you." You'll discover that sometimes all you or your partner needs is to know that you're there for each other.

As you'll see in chapters 4 and 5, helping each other to explore, address, and even heal such concerns can be exceptionally intimate and truly profound. Supporting one another in working through a fear that's holding one of you back, assisting each other in making a breakthrough in how you see yourselves, or encouraging each other to fully open up to your capacity for pleasure is deeply gratifying. Because of the enhanced intimacy that such moments foster, some couples say they go on to have the most intensely loving sex they've ever experienced.

REMEMBER THE TSUNAMI

Multiple studies have confirmed that the more gratitude you have for your partner and the more often you express it, the happier you both will feel about being together. So spend some time contemplating all the contributions your partner has made to your life. You might even find appreciation for some of the more challenging aspects of your relationship. As much as we might resist them, it's often through those challenges that we grow the most. Also make it a practice to express your gratitude often. Expressing gratitude increases both your awareness of all that's good in the life you have together and the feelings of intimacy and love between you. When someone validates you for just being in their life and being who you are, it naturally draws you closer to them.

As for your sex life, even if you're not yet having all the experiences you'd like, appreciate whatever adventures you *have* had together and whatever activities your partner *is* up for. Even though true appreciation isn't about manipulation, you may well discover that appreciation can have the delightful side effect of making your desired future experiences more likely to happen.

Cultivating gratitude for your partner is also an effective way of cultivating desire for them. This is especially helpful to know if your lives are so full with work and family obligations that you just don't have much opportunity for intimacy until the end of the day, when you're both worn out. A little gratitude here and there ("I really appreciated your help with that today." "This tastes really good. Thank you for making it!") can give you a little energy lift for enjoying a few sweet moments together later, whether that's sneaking outside while the kids are occupied to share a kiss under the stars or just falling asleep in each other's arms.

You can make plans with the best of intentions, assuming that you will both still be here tomorrow, next week, next month, or next year—*but you can never be sure*. When a tsunami hits, there's often very little warning. Families and homes can be wiped out in a matter of minutes, turning communities upside down and leaving lives forever changed. We don't know when it will happen, we don't know what form it will take, but the tsunami—or the hurricane, the fire, the financial crisis, the illness—is going to come. People who are facing their own death often suddenly and profoundly comprehend the preciousness of life and the limited time they have left with those they love. Remind yourself that the end is one breath away and that your relationship as you know it could be over in a flash and will, beyond doubt, end eventually. That acknowledgment keeps you in touch with what's important in each moment and helps you make the most of every experience you have together.

Life is short, love is sweet, and connection is everything. Love as if the tsunami is coming, because in one form or another, it is. Your time together, no matter how long or how short, is precious. If you've found someone willing to stretch into life with you, to take a little risk, to explore and keep your connection evolving and deepening, you've found someone to be truly grateful for.

3

EROTIC VERSATILITY: DIMENSIONS OF SEXUAL CONNECTION

Avery has always approached sex as an entirely physical pursuit. For Avery, sex is about sensations, physical pleasure, and orgasms. Avery's most memorable and meaningful sexual experiences involve a feeling of being physically united as one.

For Devon, sex is a creative, exciting adventure. Devon's always up for trying something new, acting out sexy scenarios and fantasies, and conjuring up one-of-a-kind sexual adventures.

Then there's Kris. For Kris, the allure of sex is its heart-opening qualities. Sex for Kris is all about connecting emotionally, feeling safe to be vulnerable and open, and sharing one's innermost feelings and desires.

Maybe you're already familiar with these three dimensions of sexual connection: sex as a physical experience, sex as a creative adventure, and sex as an expression of emotional connection. If you're like most people, one or perhaps two of these dimensions feel most familiar or meaningful to you.

Someone's dominant sexual dimension may be, in part, a response to childhood experiences. A child who grew up learning that sexuality is an expression of love and affection might, as an adult, associate sex with love, romance, and emotional intimacy. Early or frequent exposure to pornography could lead someone to develop a more physical orientation to sexuality, as porn can be limited in its portrayal of intimacy. Our initial sexual experiences and relationships can also be influential. If one's first lover was more experienced, for example, and showed them how much fun imagination and creativity could be in the bedroom, they might be inclined to approach future partners with a sense of playfulness and adventure.

Being drawn more to one dimension than another can also just be a reflection of one's individual nature or personality. Someone who has an active mind may naturally take a more creative approach to sexuality, while connecting on an emotional level doesn't come that easily to them. Someone who was raised in an environment where the topic of sex was steeped in shame or fear might find that no dimension feels particularly appealing to them.

Now let's imagine that any two of these three individuals—Avery, Devon, or Kris—meet and start dating. When people have strong preferences for different dimensions, they may feel they're never quite syncing up sexually. Although they might be well matched in other ways, if one is primarily attracted to the physical dimension, for example, and the other is all about emotional connection, that disparity could eventually leave them both feeling frustrated and unfulfilled. The sexual aspect of their relationship is unlikely to be satisfying over the long term for either of them—that is, unless one or both are willing to explore the other's primary or preferred style of sexual expression.

While having different dominant dimensions *could* make it difficult for two people to connect sexually, it's just as possible for that difference to contribute greatly to their sexual connection. If they're both willing to open up to their partner's preferred dimension, and to be their partner's loving and supportive guide into their own, those shared explorations will be extraordinarily intimate. And the perspectives and strengths they each have to offer will undoubtedly enrich their sexual engagement over time.

Even when people share an interest in the same dimension, if they never evolve—either by going more deeply into what they already share or exploring another dimension together—their sex life may one day start to feel routine or stagnant. Like the couple who enjoys doing it in the shower every Sunday morning, repetition and routine can be quite satisfying. But injecting some variety into their sex life will ensure that it never becomes mundane and they continue to look forward to their special weekend ritual.

It's helpful to recognize that these three major arenas of sexual connection correspond to three fundamental aspects of the human experience: physical (body), intellectual/creative (mind), and emotional (heart). One dimension is no better than any other, and someone having a preference for any of them doesn't mean they are doing sex "wrong." A deep sense of connection is possible through any of the three, and each can feel profoundly meaningful.

Finally, there's the spiritual dimension, which many people believe is the fourth aspect of the human experience, as in "body, mind, heart, and soul." It's interesting that when people speak of sexual experiences that they felt had a soulful or spiritual aspect to them, they often got there through one or more of the other dimensions. Rather than being *separate* from the other dimensions, soulfulness is a quality of experience that is often accessed *through* those other dimensions. There are people for whom the notion of a spiritual dimension of sexuality just sounds too "out there." However, they may be able to appreciate the idea of an experience that's so all-encompassing or profound that they would feel comfortable calling it a transformative or "peak" sexual experience. We'll explore all of this in more depth later.

If you're missing out on any of the sexual dimensions, you're also missing out on opportunities for intimacy. By opening yourself to all the dimensions of sexual connection, you'll be a more versatile lover. And you'll never run out of ways to keep your erotic connection fully charged.

THE PHYSICAL DIMENSION: FLESHLY DELIGHTS

When we hear the word *sex*, most of us probably picture naked bodies engaged in specific physical acts. Virtually all mainstream pornography also focuses on the physical aspects of sex, on stimulating certain body parts in certain ways, with penetration and orgasm as the ultimate goal. But there's so much more to explore in the physical arena of sexuality than the handful of sex acts we've given names to. There's an entire world of sensation and sensuality! To take just one example, how many different ways can you think of to tease a nipple erect? And how many of those are regularly shown in porn?

If you're someone for whom the physical dimension of sexuality seems the least important, remember that touching, hugging, and kissing have all been proven to be good for your health. Besides giving you feelings of pleasure and maybe even a sense of euphoria, some of the hormones that get stirred up during physical intimacy not only promote empathy and communication, but also ease depression and stress. Orgasms can help the heart, the prostate, the pelvic floor, and the immune system stay healthy and strong. And by having more of them, you might very well be more energetic, feel younger, and live longer.[1]

Practice ESP: Erotic Sensory Perception

One way to immerse yourself more fully in the physical dimension of sexuality is by learning to appreciate your body, whatever its age, shape, or size, as a sensual, erotic instrument. As children, we're naturally sensual, delighting in a world filled with textures, tastes, shapes, and sensations. In the process of growing up, we often lose this sensual intimacy with our surroundings. We're taught to shift our focus from what we're experiencing through our senses to what we are thinking with our minds, to be more concerned with how we look from the outside than with how we feel on the inside. Another contributor to this sensual disconnection is *sensory adaptation*, or becoming less and less responsive to the same stimulus over time. This function of your body's sensory systems is essential, as it keeps you from being distracted by the traffic outside your window when you're concentrating on work, among other things. Any unimportant sensory input is ignored so that we can maintain focus on what's most important at any given moment, including meeting our survival needs.

The trouble is, when you're making love, the input your senses are receiving is very important. You *want* to fully experience your lover's kiss. You *want* to notice when their breathing changes in response to your touch. You *want* to see the sparkle in their eyes, even when you've looked into them a thousand times before.

You can counter this tendency to become less and less attuned to your senses through an easy sensual awareness practice. Simply pay a little more attention to any pleasurable sensory experiences you happen to be having at the moment. When you sit down to a meal and take that first bite, briefly close your eyes and allow the flavors to come alive in your mouth. If you're out for a walk, notice the feeling of your body in motion, the air against your skin, and the sights, smells, and sounds around you. When you're listening to music, really tune into the voices and instruments, the melodies and harmonies; feel the rhythms moving through your body. Wherever you find yourself, allow yourself a minute to look around and take in all the colors, patterns, shapes, and shadows you see.

If you're a busy person who's thinking, *Who has time for this?*, these practices are perfect for you, as they require no extra time at all! And tuning into your senses throughout the day keeps them turned on, making it a little easier to get into the mood and feel sexually alive and responsive.

Indulging in some solo sensual eroticism is another way to cultivate sensory awareness. When you're showering, luxuriate in the feeling of being warm and wet, of soaping up your body, of toweling yourself dry. Wear underwear that makes you feel sexy, or go without because the secret exposure is freeing or feels a little naughty—in a good way. When you're stretching or exercising, notice the sensual feeling of movement and your muscles tightening and relaxing. Lie in bed and run your hands over your body, squeezing your thighs, butt, and stomach and teasing your nipples erect. And try masturbating as a purely sensory exploration. Enjoy the feeling of being turned on without trying to get off.

Come to Your Senses

When you bring these sensory awareness practices into the bedroom, sex becomes a richer experience. Look at your lover as you would a nude painting or statue. Allow your eyes to linger on their facial features, to admire the shape of their arms and legs, to see their body as a living work of art. Breathe in the smell of their hair, their skin, their breath. Taste their uniquely personal flavors. Really listen to their voice, their breathing, their moans of pleasure. Close your eyes as you run your hands over a part of their body you know well. The more attention you give to it, the more unfamiliar it will feel.

Consciously bring your awareness back to your senses whenever you notice that your mind is wandering. Remind yourself that your meeting tomorrow, the kids' schedules, and the state of politics are all irrelevant right now, and shift your attention back to the sensations your body is experiencing. This is especially valuable if you only have a brief period to be intimate, as quieting your mind will seem to stretch out the time you do have. Take in the warmth of your lover's neck, the feeling of their touch, the glistening beads of sweat on their skin, the sensuous curve of a shoulder, a cheek, a hip. By becoming more present to what's happening now, you will experience not only an increase in sensation and pleasure, but also in the degree of connection you feel.

Even hugs can be sensually connecting. When you have a few extra minutes for an extended hug, allow yourselves to fully relax into the embrace and each other. If hugging this way doesn't come naturally to you but you're open to a little experimentation, start with hugs that are just a second or two longer than usual. As you begin to soften into each other, allow any feelings of hesitation or resistance to melt away. As thoughts come up, let them drift away as well. Begin to relax any areas, such as your shoulders or neck, that don't need to be engaged for you to feel balanced, supported by your partner, and supporting of them. Scan your body for any areas you're holding away from your partner, like your chest, belly, or hips. Breathe into those areas, consciously relaxing them as you exhale. The more you let go, the more you will encourage your partner to also let go. Allow yourself to really experience holding your lover and being held by them. Feel your connection everywhere your bodies touch. Feel the warmth and aliveness of your bodies as you luxuriate in the sweet feelings stirred up through a long hug.

When you kiss your lover's shoulder, feel the warmth of the skin through your lips. As you press your mouth into that feeling, breathe in the scent of their skin. When your mouths touch, let your lips and tongue be curious, playful, receptive, enjoying the erotic energy, the tastes, the sensations. Have no agenda here, no idea of what kissing is supposed to be like. Let the kiss be created by the two of you right there in that moment. Experiment with different places to kiss. How about on a staircase or in the shower? Or get totally into however your partner is kissing. Even if you've kissed like that a thousand times before, you'll be surprised how newly intimate their kiss can feel.

Maintain your sensory connection with each other during vaginal or anal penetration by being aware of all the sensations you're feeling: flesh against warm flesh, the weight of your bodies pressing together, the mesmerizing movements, the rhythmic slapping or slippery wet sounds, the intensifying stimulation in your genitals. Notice the sensations created by various positions, angles of penetration, and tempos. And enjoy all the visual pleasures of your bodies moving together, which can be a tremendous turn-on.

Oral Eroticism

Of all the ways sex gives us to revel in our senses, there is perhaps no sex act more filled with sensual possibility than oral sex. "You're right up in the most vulnerable area of his body, so there's this incredible level of trust—you've got teeth!" laughs Jody. "There's also this very sensitive barometer in your mouth that tells you exactly what's getting him excited. You can feel the blood rushing and smell the masculine scents that start to rise when a man is turned on."

To many people, oral sex can feel more physically intimate than intercourse: "Holding her hips in my hands, exploring her with my mouth and tongue, seeing her swell in response to my attention is the most intimate form of connection," Frankie says.

While it's certainly possible to have a satisfying sex life without oral sex—and many couples do—it's just as true that a couple who doesn't engage in oral sex may be missing out on opportunities for sensual exploration and pleasure. This is especially true for women who don't generally climax through vaginal penetration (which is the majority), since cunnilingus may be their easiest avenue to not only arousal, but also to orgasm.

Some people shy away from oral sex because of ideas like only certain kinds of people do that, which is absolutely untrue—all kinds of people do that. Others are afraid that it's not clean. If that's your fear, and there's not time to enjoy a sexy shower together, there's always a warm washcloth. And if your partner's personal hygiene is good, remember that the smells their body produces when sexually aroused are meant to be natural aphrodisiacs. If you're afraid your lover won't be turned on by how you smell, taste, or look or by how you're responding to their attention, having some "oral sex" around oral sex—in other words, talking about it—will help you lay those fears to rest.

Another consideration is that countless women are emerging from hookup culture feeling uncomfortable about receiving pleasure, asking for what they want, or even knowing what they want. Study after study confirms that men are more likely than women to receive oral sex during a heterosexual hookup.[2] It's not uncommon for men to expect oral sex but be reluctant or unwilling to reciprocate. "Guys have told me they won't go down on a girl if they're just hooking up, only if they get to know her," says Clara, a fourth-year college student. "But they definitely have an expectation that the woman will go down on them. Guys know it's more difficult for women to orgasm, so they often use that as an excuse to not even try." If a woman hasn't yet been with a lover who appreciates this delightfully pleasurable act of intimacy, it's no wonder she might be uncomfortable about receiving!

Still other people have had traumatic experiences with oral sex or feel it makes them too vulnerable or puts them in a place of subjugation. In these instances, talking things over with a counselor can be helpful, as can the magnificently intimate experience of exploring these challenges with a supportive partner, as we cover in chapters 4 and 5.

In a lot of mainstream pornography, scenes involving fellatio and cunnilingus tend to be fairly predictable and limited. Actors might jump right into full-on oral sex with no buildup at all. This is unfortunate, because oral sex is a perfect opportunity to set your sensual creativity free. Next time, try imagining that your partner's genitals start at their toes and work your way up, or at their ears and work your way down. You might inquire what kind of touch they would like you to begin with, whether that's kissing, cuddling, licking, or massage—all of which can bring blood to the area, increasing their arousal and having them craving more direct stimulation.

Most porn would also have us believe that all fellatio should be performed on an erect penis. But there's so much eroticism and pleasure to be had during the transition from soft to hard. "It's super sensual to feel yourself becoming erect in your partner's mouth," says Derek. "Moving from one state to the other feels unbelievably sensuous."

Erections come and go and come back again quite naturally during sex, especially during longer sessions of play and exploration, and that doesn't mean it's not erotic and enjoyable or that something is going wrong. There's so much expectation around getting hard at the "right" times, and shame when things don't go according to plan. Yet playing with all the different states of erection can be pleasurable for both the giver and the receiver. Remember, a soft penis has the same number of nerve endings as a hard one! People can also feel the expectation or pressure to ejaculate during certain activities, and embarrassment if that's not what's happening for them. For anyone who experiences difficulty getting or maintaining an erection—or reaching orgasm, for that matter—a partner who is willing to treat oral play as an occasion for eroticism and connection can be a dream come true.

Though there are plenty of techniques to experiment with, the ultimate secret to giving great oral sex is to *enjoy it*. When you're totally into it, indulging in all of the textures and tastes and rhythms, and listening with all of your senses to your partner's responses, you'll be creating your own "techniques" in the moment. And be playful!

When you discover something your lover really likes—maybe a special trick you do with your tongue—give it a name to help you both remember it: "Ooo, I'd love it if you'd do your double spiral maneuver right about now!"

Just like fellatio, the best, most delicious cunnilingus is when you're really connecting with your lover's feel, smell, and taste, and all the lovely curves and textures. Don't rush over any one part to get to another. If you move too fast or go for the more sensitive areas too quickly, your partner won't be able to fully relax and will likely be tensing their muscles to protect themselves. Take time to appreciate how the outer lips differ from the inner lips, how sensual it feels to move your tongue between and around them. Stay tuned into your lover's body for signs of arousal: their breath deepening, their thighs relaxing, their pelvis arching toward you, their labia and clitoris swelling, and any sounds of pleasure they're making.

One more tip we can't emphasize enough: don't leave pleasure to find pleasure. If she's getting into something you're doing, *keep doing it*! "Typically a lover will do something for ten or twenty seconds, and then speed up or move to something else," says Katerina. "But if they're doing something I'm enjoying and they just stay there and keep doing that, in ten minutes I'll be going out of my mind!" If your lover knows you'll be there for a while, they can just let go and fully indulge themselves in the sensations you're creating.

Here's a sensory awareness practice you can try together: orally pleasuring each other at the same time while putting all of your attention on your senses. If you're one of the many people who find "69" distracting because it's difficult to concentrate on being both the giver and the receiver at once, this suggestion is for you! Find a position that's comfortable for you both (supportive pillows can help) and then focus your awareness on all your senses. If distracting thoughts come up (like, "This has never worked for me. Why would it work now?"), let them go by turning your attention back to the sensations you're experiencing, including the tactile delights of your hands, mouths, arms, and legs intertwining in this intimate way. Orgasms aren't the goal here—physical connection and sensual pleasure are. Imagine that you're channeling the pleasurable feelings you're receiving back into those you're offering. When you're able to be completely present to both the pleasure you're giving and the pleasure you're receiving, you will feel a shift from this being two separate acts you're engaged in to one intensely intimate experience. You might even notice a current of erotic energy circulating between you. Really, you just might!

So yes, it's certainly possible for two people to have a satisfying sex life without engaging in oral sex. But once they experience its endless potential for intimacy and sensual pleasure, it's highly unlikely they'll want to!

THE CREATIVE DIMENSION: THE ART OF ADVENTURE

Let's turn next to the creative, adventurous dimension of sexuality. Most new relationships offer a sense of adventure just by virtue of being new. There's simply no "same old thing" you can do—yet. It's not uncommon for couples to be quite sexually creative when they're first together and then, after a few months—or, if they're lucky, a few years—they stop experimenting and eventually find themselves just going through the motions. Sex may become so predictable that some nights it doesn't even feel worth the effort it takes for an orgasm. But just having a willingness to try something new, to be inventive and imaginative, can be enough to keep sexual stagnation at bay. When you tap into the creative dimension, you'll discover that there are a million ways to make love.

The creative dimension of sexuality can be particularly compelling for people with very active minds. If their mind is not involved in the experience they're having, it will often wander off in search of something else to do, like reviewing the details of yesterday's interaction at work or making plans for the upcoming weekend, which takes them out of the present moment. Actively involving their mind in lovemaking gives it something to do that contributes to the experience rather than detracting from it.

Creativity can be intentional and deliberate. You could design an entire experience in advance, like gifting your lover with an evening at their own personal "sex spa." There are so many possibilities in just this one scenario. Prepare the bathroom with candles and music, offer your "client" a glass of champagne, treat them to a foot scrub and massage, or decorate them with body paints and then take photos of your sensual artwork. Then present them with a menu of your sexual services. Give this last one some thought. What would be on *your* menu of services? And don't forget the Daily Special!

There are also spontaneous acts of creativity: touching the ice cube you're holding in your mouth to your lover's neck, catching their eye from across the room as you bite delicately into a strawberry, or squeezing their thigh under the table when you're out with friends in a way that says "I want this later!"

Try using a creative intention to embellish oral sex. For instance, imagine that this is the very first time you've ever gone down on your lover or that they haven't been orally pleasured in years and you're here to right that wrong. One time, make it as sweet as you possibly can. Another time, ask them to direct you verbally while you do exactly as they tell you. Or put on some of their favorite music and pretend they're an instrument you're playing or that they are your mouth's dance partner. If this sounds silly, we hope we can persuade you to give it a try anyway. It can be such rhythmic, sensual fun!

Fantasy Play

Perhaps the most obvious, and certainly limitless, area of sexual creativity is fantasy play. Trying on new personas takes us beyond our usual patterns and perceptions of ourselves. Sex therapist David Schnarch says the great benefit of role-playing is that it "permits unmatched sexual variety (and meaningful engagement) *with the same person* over a lifetime."[3]

If play-acting in the bedroom seems too contrived to you, let's not forget that sex can also be fun! You don't have to be a professional actor, and you don't need elaborate dialogue or scenarios. In fact, just the offhand suggestion of a role, like, "Oh, are you my new personal trainer?" or "Those glasses make you look like a college professor I'd like to seduce!" can jump-start a session of sexy playtime. It might also help to know that in a study of 70,000 people, one out of four of those who described their relationship as extremely sexually satisfying said that they incorporated role-play into their sex lives.[4] Besides, being able to relax your inhibitions—which pretending to be someone else might require you to do—is among the most useful sexual skills you will ever develop.

If you resist the idea of fantasy play because you feel it's inauthentic, know that it feels more authentic the more you immerse yourselves in the personas you're taking on. It truly can feel like you're interacting as two new people. And that's exciting!

One of our most memorable sexual encounters was the time I (Mali) was visited by a charismatic alien from outer space while Joe and I were camping. He entered the tent, whispered to me not to be afraid, and explained that he'd been sent to this planet to conduct a thorough inspection of a female Earthling. Being an avid Star Trek fan, this close encounter felt almost destined to happen to me one day. We spent the next two hours taking sexual exploration to the outer limits while laughing ourselves crazy.

Then there was the night I (Joe) was "hired" to be Mali's escort for the evening. We started our date by traveling separately to a candlelit Spanish restaurant. The couple at the next table spent their entire meal trying to covertly listen in on our conversation, which included fabricated tales of other "clients" I'd had and Mali's encounters with previous "service providers." After two hours of this erotic charade, I was so turned on that all I wanted to do was follow my benefactor back to her place and let her have her way with me!

Yes, it can feel a bit silly to play an extraterrestrial or an experienced gigolo, but playfulness around sex is invigorating. And allowing yourselves to let go once in a while means you can have a new erotic adventure anytime.

Testing the Waters

Your most personal source of new ideas to experiment with is, of course, your own sexual interests, turn-ons, and fantasies. But because we humans have so many fears, insecurities, judgments, and misconceptions tangled up with sex, revealing our interests to each other is best done with thoughtfulness and sensitivity. This is especially true if those interests seem far from the mainstream.

The fact that people's histories, beliefs, and attitudes around sexuality are so diverse means there is no advice we can offer that will cover every situation. But we believe the following ideas will be helpful.

People can have wildly different reactions to hearing about their partner's sexual fantasies. Some people would be receptive to almost any fantasy their lover might have. Yvonne, in her late twenties, says, "If I like a guy, learning about some fantasy he has doesn't change who he is. Besides, his fantasies are useful to me, because they turn him on." But what if he actually wants to dress up in your underwear? "I'd be happy to sacrifice a few of my panties for the cause," she laughs, "as long as he takes me shopping for new ones!"

Other people, especially those for whom sex is primarily about emotional connection, might feel uncomfortable with the idea that their partner even has fantasies. Catherine and Josh, for example, have been together for fifteen years, and both say they have a satisfying sex life. But Catherine believes that if Josh were truly satisfied, he wouldn't have a need to fantasize. Josh has reassured Catherine that having an occasional fantasy doesn't mean he isn't attracted to her or doesn't love her. But she is adamant that people who are in love should never fantasize. Now, it's possible that Catherine is one of the approximately 3 percent of people who don't ever have sexual fantasies, so the concept just doesn't make sense to her.[5] Or maybe she does have them occasionally, but they make her feel uncomfortable or ashamed. Or she might believe that if a person has a fantasy, it means they necessarily want to make that fantasy happen in reality—that there's no such thing as fantasizing just for fun. (For the record, having a fantasy about something does not mean that someone necessarily wants to experience that something in reality.) Whatever the reasons for Catherine's discomfort with the idea of her husband's erotic imaginings, Josh made a choice years ago to avoid any discussion with Catherine about the topic. Unfortunately, Josh's decision might actually lessen the couple's potential for intimacy. And it is intimacy that Catherine craves most of all.

For many couples, letting each other in on a fantasy, and even playing with one together, is an inventive way to spend an evening. There may be some advance preparation to do, however, to get to a place where sharing and playing with fantasies together is a possibility for you. Getting comfortable talking about sex in general, and diverse sexual interests in particular, will help you gauge just how receptive your partner might be to hearing about *your* fantasies and interests.

If you and your partner are not already in the habit of sharing your sexual interests and fantasies but are intrigued by the prospect, the following ideas will help you overcome obstacles that might be in the way and build trust between you in the process. Even if you never reveal your deepest desires to each other, just moving in that direction will open up new opportunities for intimacy and keep your relationship erotically charged.

You could begin by talking about sexual interests in a general way, exploring questions like these:

- What are some wild or unusual sexual practices you've heard of? (This is all relative, of course. Being spanked or blindfolded or having sex in a public place, for example, would seem quite unusual to some people and not at all to others.)
- What would either of us think if the other actually had one of those interests? Would we want to know about it?

Expand on this conversation by exploring specific interests some people have, such as voyeurism (arousal through watching others) and exhibitionism (arousal through being watched). You may never have thought of yourself as either a voyeur or an exhibitionist, but millions of people find some version of these interests quite compelling. Put aside the more extreme examples, like people who peer into their neighbor's windows or expose themselves to strangers, and consider the number of people who regularly post sexy photos of themselves and the number who take pleasure in viewing those images. We predict that you, too, have at least a touch of the voyeur or exhibitionist in you. Have you ever been turned on watching a lover shower, exercise, dance, or sleep? Have you enjoyed being watched by them? Try playing with a little voyeurism and exhibitionism together. Observe through the window as your partner undresses. Let your lover relax back into a chair while you dance seductively or touch yourself for their viewing pleasure. Or enjoy the reflections of your intertwined bodies making passionate love in a mirror you've positioned just right.

You can see that you don't have to be into a particular turn-on yourselves to be inspired by it. There are hundreds of recognized sexual interests, or what psychologists call paraphilias, that could spark some provocative "oral sex." You can spend hours indulging your imaginations together and talking about the many varied and crazy things that we humans are into.

It's important to note that we're discussing paraphilic *desires* here rather than the far more serious paraphilic *disorders*. A sexual interest is considered a disorder if the person is hurting someone (or something) or if that interest has created a pattern of distress for them.[6]

That said, how might you two incorporate a little pygophilia (arousal by the human derrière) into your next erotic encounter? In other words, what might you do if you had a passion for asses? Suggest your lover wear something that you particularly enjoy seeing them in—from behind. Steal a moment here and there to run your fingers over their curves. When you embrace, let your hands wander downwards and explore. You might even invite them to experience a sensuous session of ass-worshiping. Have some lotion or oil handy and help them get comfortable lying face down, supporting their hips with a pillow or two. Now, start slowly. You are a pygophiliac, and you want to savor this experience! Immerse yourself in caressing, stroking, squeezing, and kissing their flesh. Invite them to tell you what they like and what they don't, and especially what they'd like more of. If they're up for it, experiment with more stimulating kinds of touch. Start slowly with sexy nibbles, playful pinches, or light slaps, paying attention to their responses and letting any sighs, moans, or movements guide you. This could make for arousing foreplay if you're already into anal play, and a sexy introduction if you haven't yet explored it.

Now that you get the idea, how might you explore some knismophilia (arousal through tickling or being tickled)? What fun might you have if you were a pair of pictophiliacs (aroused by erotic art) or xylophiliacs (aroused by wood)? Be a little adventurous, and you might never look at your kitchen table in the same way again. And if you're wondering if desires like these are really a thing, the answer is yes, most certainly—as is probably everything else you can possibly think of!

Conversations and playful attitudes around topics like these will help you get a sense of whether either of you might be receptive to revealing or hearing about any of your *own* interests. For example, if your partner has a negative reaction to something you're actually interested in, that's good information to have before you open up about it. On the other hand, if you happen to come across something about which you both say, "I'd be up for trying this," that's even better information!

Another potentially enlightening topic is fantasies and desires you had when you were younger: *What sensual or erotic thoughts can you remember having when you were younger? How did you feel about those thoughts at the time? Where or how might those ideas or images have originated?* Some people will remember fantasies that are quite elaborate or complex, while others may recall only subtle or fleeting impressions. Either way, these conversations can be both revealing and insightful. Discovering any connections to the present can also be fascinating: *Are there any ways those erotic ideas are reflected in who you are today?*

You might also explore fantasies either of you has that are entirely beyond the realm of possibility, like having sex with a centaur or being a concubine in ancient Japan. Because they're unattainable, fantasies like these are less likely to trigger a partner's fears or insecurities.[7]

Sharing Your Sexual Interests

Justin Lehmiller, social psychologist and author of *Tell Me What You Want: The Science of Sexual Desire and How It Can Help You Improve Your Sex Life*, surveyed over 4000 people about their sexual fantasies. Most of the respondents had positive experiences sharing their fantasies with a partner. He offers these tips for success: Build trust and intimacy first (hopefully, you've been doing that!). Choose a quiet, private place, and perhaps wait until the two of you are already turned on, as your partner might be more receptive at that time. And reassure your partner that you love the sex life you have together and just want to add something to it.[8]

If you open up about a turn-on, ease into it. Suppose you have a desire to be dominated sexually, an exceedingly common sexual interest. You might say, "Every once in a while, I imagine you telling me exactly what you want me to do to you" or "I've sometimes fantasized about you blindfolding me and tying my hands to the bed while you explore my body." Share with your lover why these ideas excite you. Maybe they give you an intense feeling of being desired, or there's a sense of freedom in letting go and surrendering to the will of the person you love and trust the most.

Don't be attached to the idea of your partner enthusiastically jumping right in to make all your dreams come true. It could take many conversations, and fantasizing together, before something happens, if it ever does. Even if your explorations never move beyond the verbal, these interactions can go a long way toward satisfying that desire while bonding you in a very intimate way.

If your partner reveals one of their interests to you, remember that although anything you've not considered before might make you feel a little uncomfortable, their interests are windows into their erotic imagination. So listen with receptivity and nonjudgment. In finally being able to safely share this secret, which they may have kept hidden for years, your lover may feel both relieved and grateful.

"I'm really sensitive to this," says Morgan, "as I've been with lovers who have suffered with the belief that they are very weird or their desires are weird. And often they're *so* not weird at all and super common, but they've just never revealed them before and have lived with such crippling shame. Even though it was hard to understand how things had evolved for them to feel that way, their pain was real."

You can encourage your lover to open up more with questions like these: *Can you remember anything about your earliest experiences with this desire? How has it evolved over time? How does this fantasy make you feel? Could you describe for me one scenario you've imagined? How does it feel to share this with me?* Read some articles or stories about the topic together, and you'll no doubt discover that there are countless other people out there with the exact same interest.

Why say yes to exploring your lover's desires with them? People whose partners are willing to indulge their desires report being more satisfied with their relationship and more committed to its success. And those doing the indulging say that finding ways to share in their partner's interests makes them feel good about themselves and their relationship.[9] Besides, the thrill of seeing your lover really turned on can lead to super-hot sex!

I (Mali) have personal experience with this. Soon after we met, my college boyfriend casually mentioned that he thought underarm hair on a woman was sexy. At first I was shocked. This was certainly not what I'd been raised to see as attractive! Despite my strong feelings, I kept thinking about it. I knew that my feeling of revulsion was a learned cultural response—there was nothing "gross" or "unhygienic" about underarm hair. Certainly men didn't have these labels applied to *their* body hair! I kept talking to my boyfriend about it, who, of course, had also grown up being told that female body hair was unacceptable. In fact, this probably contributed to his attraction. In his mind, unshaved underarms on a female were transgressive—a violation of socially acceptable norms—and a reminder of a woman's wild, animal nature.

It was summer and we were living in Berkeley, California, a city known around the world for being socially liberal. If there were ever a time and place for this walk on the wild side, this was it. I would blend right in! I finally accepted that I had no good answer to his question, "What would be the harm in not shaving under your arms for a while?" So for two months I went au naturel, and he absolutely loved it. He made me feel incredibly hot and was abundantly grateful! I liked that I was getting over my culturally learned distaste and that, even in that short time span, eventually I rarely ever thought about it. I was proud of myself for giving it a try, and I'm happy that today women everywhere are defying this and other restrictive beauty standards, despite the criticism and extreme reactions they often have to put up with. It's also fascinating that one of the functions of underarm hair is to convey pheromones, those olfactory sexual attractants, and that the smell of one's lover can be an unparalleled turn-on in part because of them!

There are almost always ways to indulge each other's desires that you will both feel good about. Suppose that many years into their relationship, Patrick admits to Lucy that he sometimes has hotwife fantasies, in which he envisions Lucy having sex with another man. This is another extremely common desire, with thousands of websites devoted to it.[10] Like every sexual desire, denying that it exists won't make it go away. Even if Lucy is certain she would never be interested in actually playing out this scenario, there are still ways this couple could explore it together. They could watch movies or read erotic stories about the topic, talk about it while they're having sex as an extra turn-on, or role-play some scenarios. To make all of this a possibility for Lucy, Patrick, of course, will need to resist pressuring her to take their explorations into real life.

As another example, suppose Lucy reveals that she's turned on by the idea of having sex in public, but Patrick (despite his hotwife fantasies) is unnerved by the possibility of actually getting caught. They could still have fun searching for places where the likelihood of actually being discovered is quite low—in the window of a room in a large hotel; in a remote, secluded area outdoors; or in a car parked down a deserted road.

One reason someone might be reluctant to explore their partner's interest is the fear that their partner will then want to do it all the time. But if you're having lots of other connecting sexual experiences, a new addition to your erotic repertoire is unlikely to suddenly take over your entire sex life. If this is your partner's fear, it's up to you to make sure it's not a valid one!

With open minds and a little creativity, you and your lover's sexual interests, turn-ons, and fantasies can be an endless source of sexy inspiration and erotic connection. How cool is that?

Here's one more compelling reason to develop sexual creativity. When you're together for the long term, you'll inevitably experience changes and challenges in your lives, your bodies, and your libidos. Navigating these changes in a way that keeps your connection solid and your sex life compelling and fun is much easier when you're open-minded, curious—and creative!

THE EMOTIONAL DIMENSION: TOUCHING THE HEART

The third and perhaps most underrated dimension of sexual connection is the emotional dimension. For people whose most profound sexual experiences involve feelings of deep intimacy, caring, and heartfelt communication, connecting emotionally makes sex much more meaningful and satisfying.

"For me, it's the difference between having sex and making love," explains Kelly, a self-described demisexual, or person who doesn't experience sexual attraction in the absence of an emotional connection. "Having just a physical experience leaves me feeling hollow."

"A strong emotional bond with someone who loves and accepts me helps me feel safe to fully let go," Courtney says. "And the orgasms I have with someone who totally and completely accepts me are unlike any other. Otherwise so many thoughts are in the background, holding me back: 'Oh, I'm taking too long, they'll get bored.' 'I should come a certain way, it should look a certain way, I should sound a certain way.'"

"Emotional connection is at the heart of passion," says Rod. "Without passion, sex is just exercise." And Ethan says that when he's out of a relationship, one of the things he misses most is kissing: "It's the connection I crave. I can get the physical release through masturbation." Veteran sex therapist Marty Klein agrees. "When adults experience passion, it's usually not in response to incredible sex or the perfect body," he says. "It's usually in response to giving themselves permission to let go emotionally."[11]

Without an emotional dimension, even a relationship that's intended to be purely sexual can soon begin to feel like it's missing something. In the college hookup culture, where people regularly engage in one-night stands or ongoing sex-only relationships, both women and men speak of having to work hard not to form emotional attachments to the people they're getting together with. Yet it's precisely because of the lack of emotional connection, they say, that they can find these experiences superficial and ultimately unfulfilling.[12] The wise sex therapist Jack Morin offers a simple but profound explanation for this: "Feelings," he says, "make sex matter."[13]

Even when a committed couple does continue to have regular sex, if they start to lose touch with their emotional connection, or never felt much of one from the start, their relationship might eventually feel as though it lacks romance, passion, and depth. For us, although we both love the physicality of sex, even our most intense physical experiences are also an expression of—and profoundly enhanced by—our emotional connection.

For some, an emotional connection is essential for experiencing sexual pleasure. Maya, for instance, has always felt vulnerable during oral sex. "When Kim is way down there, the distance is uncomfortable," she says. "We've discovered that we can create a 'bridge of connection' through eye contact. I feel a sense of safety, of being held, by looking into her eyes at the same time."

It's worth mentioning here that people of all genders are interested in emotional connection. This is despite the fact that males in many cultures are often not encouraged to develop, value, or recognize their own need for emotional closeness, which can take a great toll on their relationships.[14] If you're a male, or with a male partner, seeing the cultural conditioning that might be at play can help loosen the hold that conditioning has and open up more emotional connection between the two of you.

Two Essential Elements for Emotional Connection

One easy way to strengthen your emotional connection is through the liberal use of empathy and reassurance. These emotionally validating behaviors can have an almost magical effect in many situations. In fact, a little empathy and reassurance can sometimes make the difference between having a horrible experience and a transformational one!

Let's take a closer look at these two essential elements for emotional connection:

- **Empathy** is the ability to understand and vicariously experience someone else's feelings, thoughts, and attitudes. To become more empathetic, give your partner your full attention. Encourage them to put their experiences and emotions into words, without interrupting or offering suggestions. For a moment, imagine what it would be like to be in their situation, with their history, their experiences, and their fears. This will help you reach a place of "emotional resonance," or to feel what they are feeling. Being able to authentically say, "I can understand how you're feeling" will help them feel heard and supported.

- **Reassurance** is the action of calming someone's doubts, fears, or worries, which will help them feel safe. Reassurance can be in the form of comforting words: "I'm here for you." "We're in this together." "You're the most important person in my life." "You are more than good enough." "I'm not going anywhere." "I love you just the way you are." Reassurance can also be communicated through eye contact, a hug, or even just a squeeze of the hand.

If your partner is struggling with something—anything!—empathy and reassurance will often help them begin to relax. You can even empower each other to ask for empathy or reassurance when you could really use it.

Emotional Foreplay

A little intentional romance is another simple way to stay emotionally bonded. Back rubs, candles, and clean sheets can be enough to create a sweet sense of romance. Kiss his neck as you walk by his computer. Send a flirty text. Sensuously feed him the last bite of chocolate. Caress her cheek or hold her face in your hands. These are all effortless gestures that convey a feeling that your partner is loved, beautiful, and desirable. Check in and ask, "How are you feeling?" and really listen to the answer. Watch more sunsets. When was the last time you stood arm in arm witnessing the beauty and sacredness of the setting sun?

Before a date, intentionally reconnect with that sense of anticipation you had earlier on in your relationship. Did you do anything special to get ready, like having a bath, putting on some music, or dressing up in something that makes you feel particularly attractive? Tap into the excitement you experienced while doing these things again now. Shave with a purpose—not just because you do that five days a week, but because smooth skin will make kissing you all the more pleasurable for your partner.

As you relax into each other and into your time together, take a moment to connect by making eye contact, holding hands, or kissing. A long hug, in which you allow yourselves to fully let go and feel grounded and safe, is another easy way to heighten your awareness of the emotional connection you share.

For many people, the emotional dimension is the most vulnerable, as it requires a willingness to open up during sex. And yet the more vulnerable you are, the more potential for connection you create. Being emotionally connected while you're physically connected can make all kinds of sensual and sexual touch more meaningful and, in turn, more pleasurable. For some people, this is especially true during penetrative sex. "Being filled on the inside by someone you are crazy about is a very connecting feeling," says Ashley. "An emotional as well as a physical feeling of fullness." And Jamal says, "Being inside someone is really special. They're allowing you to experience them in one of the most physically intimate ways possible. I love wrapping myself around her while I'm inside of her and feeling her response to my presence in her."

The deep connection we humans can feel through kissing, caressing, or looking into each other's eyes during sex can make the experience more profound—even if it's just a quickie! Verbal expressions of affection or desire can also be very bonding: "Sex with you is amazing." "You're beautiful." "You're so sexy." "I love you." "I love being inside you/having you inside me."

Sometimes slowing things down can help partners stay more in touch with each other. Addison says, "A slower rhythm allows me to feel waves of sensation and connection that go far beyond the physical."

Sex therapist David Schnarch suggests that couples try having sex with their eyes open. Looking into each other's eyes while climaxing, and allowing yourselves to be fully seen, is the "epitome of intimacy," he says.[15] Feeling your emotional connection while you're looking into each other's eyes and experiencing intense pleasure is like a baring of the sexual soul.

Emotionally connected sex can be so moving that some people even experience spontaneous crying after intercourse or an orgasm. "It's an emotional release," says Jules, "and feels so cleansing."

Finally, if you've been together a while, you have the opportunity for an especially sweet level of intimacy that new couples don't yet have: you can romantically reminisce. So make the most of it! Every once in a while, play some songs the two of you listened to when you first fell in love. Reread notes you wrote to each other early on. Look through photos of special times you've had together. Celebrate the great thing you've got going by re-creating that long hug in the moonlight, holding hands at that little café, or making love in that place you've never forgotten. Look into each other's eyes and reflect on all the important life moments you've shared. Appreciate your lover for choosing to be here, now, with you.

THE SPIRITUAL DIMENSION: SEX WITH SOUL

It's probably obvious by now that the sexual dimensions are interconnected and that any one of them will enrich the others. Your creativity comes into play, for example, whenever you propose a hot new place to get physical or dream up an elaborate romantic evening. Supporting each other in trying something new or adventurous creates an abundance of emotional intimacy. And being fully present and sensually aware during lovemaking can lead to a sexual discovery that the two of you can delight in for years to come.

Countless couples have also experienced altered states of consciousness and transcendent feelings of connection during sexual experiences that involve any one or even all three of the realms we've explored so far. They describe these rare occasions as transporting them together to a place beyond the physical and even approaching what they might call the mystical, spiritual, or divine. "You meet God in sex sometimes," says our dear friend Marybeth. "Well, if it's *good* sex!" Couples sometimes talk of orgasms, too, as being a spiritual experience or a celebration of their multidimensional connection.

Other people who have had similar experiences don't think of them as spiritual and instead might refer to them as profound or "peak" experiences. In his book *Peak Sexual Experience*, psychologist John Selby says that "couples who tap into this transcendent quality of lovemaking often speak of how, each time they make love with each other, it is as if for the first time."[16]

Personal Paths to the Spiritual Dimension

So how do couples access the spiritual dimension during lovemaking? Some intentionally seek out a spiritual experience of sexuality by learning intimacy and sensuality practices such as tantra, "slow sex," and karezza (from the Italian word for "caress"). These practices are about slowing down and connecting through the entire self. They can involve breathing techniques, generous amounts of time for verbal communication, and a variety of forms of sensual touch. Couples who enjoy these practices say that setting aside time to slow down, question everything they know about sex, really feel into themselves and each other, and focus on breath, sound, and movement produces life-changing experiences. They describe an evolution in their understanding of the meaning and role of sexuality in their lives.

There's no one path to a sense of spiritual connection with your partner. The exercises we've mentioned can help some couples create that feeling. For others, such practices may seem artificial, confronting, or awkward. If that sounds like you, know that you might just be reaching a new edge. You might have more capacity to explore such realms than you previously realized—if only you can embrace a few moments of discomfort or awkwardness and allow yourself to be seen by, and to truly see, your partner.

The core ideas underlying many of these practices are themes that appear throughout this book. These themes, which are a key to creating sexual experiences that feel deeply personal and profound, are as follows:

- Slow down.
- Tune into yourself and your partner.
- Engage all of your senses.
- Give your full attention to whatever you're doing in the moment.
- Focus on feeling connection, appreciation, and acceptance and not so much on techniques and orgasms.

Couples who speak of having accessed a spiritual dimension through one or more of the other three dimensions often mention themes from the list above. For example, an intense intimacy session, in which both people feel fully desired and accepted and focus intently on the physical sensations, can cause conscious thought to fall away and produce a feeling of transcendence and euphoria.

John Selby recommends prolonging this experience by not "immediately shifting into thought mode" after sex. "As soon as we start thinking," he says, "we lose the magic of the mystic moment we have attained." Instead, "the postorgasm experience is the blessing of remaining in bliss and oneness for at least a few minutes after orgasm, enabling us to integrate this mystic experience into our everyday consciousness."[17]

Our Story: Multidimensional Lovemaking

The following story illustrates one way we have woven together our different dominant dimensions in an intensely personal and loving way that culminated in an experience that felt spiritual and transformational to us both.

We both see our emotional connection as being at the heart of our relationship. Joe's other primary dimension is the physical, while mine (Mali's) is the creative. We use this difference to our erotic advantage all the time.

Early on, during one of our many arousing and provocative conversations about sex, I asked Joe if he was a breast man, a leg man, or an ass man. His answer took me by surprise. He is, he told me, very much a pussy man. I was intrigued!

I'd never given much thought to the vulva as an object of lust and adoration. Though I didn't feel negatively about my own, I also didn't see it as particularly attractive. It occurred to me that, considering the number of women he'd made love to and the erotica he'd seen over the years (starting with the tattered copy of *Hustler* he'd managed to acquire as a young teen!), Joe had seen hundreds if not thousands of vulvas, while I'd seen relatively few.

I spent many hours over the next couple of weeks immersed in some very intimate research, sorting through thousands of photos of vulvas online. I collected several hundred pictures featuring all different shapes and skin tones and taken from various angles. When I finally let Joe know that I had an experience planned for the following weekend that would probably require a few hours, I didn't mention that what I had in mind was a private "pussyfest"!

The day arrived. We cuddled up together on the couch and I opened my computer. The look of delight that came over his face when I showed him the first image was precious. If there's one thing I love, it's seeing my guy get excited by a new sexploration!

One after another, I enlarged the photos to full screen. "So tell me, what do you appreciate about this one?" I would ask. "What do you see when you look at this?" I really wanted to understand his attraction to and appreciation for this mysterious area of the body, especially because I knew that lots of people consider their own vulva unattractive or even ugly. Joe described to me how unique and beautiful each one was and why each was, in its own way, an erotic work of art. Thick labia or thin labia, symmetrical or asymmetrical, protruding inner lips or lips that were tucked away, dark brown, caramel, pink, deep purple—I started to see that all this natural variety was captivating to him.

"What would you do if you had the opportunity to make love to this one?" I asked. "Where would you start?" In his sweet bedroom voice, Joe described to me in detail exactly what he would love to do. "Ooo, and what about *this* one?!" Joe made love to a hundred pussies that afternoon, his arms around me the entire time.

What an education I'd just had. And then, as he so often does, Joe moved us from the creative dimension into the physical. With a familiar, sexy smile, he said, "Now it's your turn."

What I saw in the small mirror he held up for me that evening was a complete shock: my vulva looked stunningly beautiful. How could I have never noticed this before? I was forty years old, and had checked myself out many times over the years. But viewing all those other vulvas through Joe's adoring eyes made me now see mine so differently. He was right. Every single one—including my own!—is a unique work of art.

Joe also took dozens of photos of me, some of them in sheer panties, others as I emerged dripping wet from the spray of the handheld shower, and I could see what he saw: every one of those images was breathtaking. I finally understood why he was so crazy about pussies, and particularly this pussy! I also discovered that night that when you learn to love your own vulva, the experience of someone else making love to it is truly indescribable.

The gift Joe gave me that weekend—a new way of seeing myself as beautiful—is still with me all these years later, as is the abundant gratitude I feel toward him for relieving me of my limiting misperceptions. Anytime I want a refresher, Joe is more than happy to oblige. I must say, he's made me very grateful to be in a relationship with a genuine pussy man!

I (Joe) learned something through this exploration too. Before that fateful evening, the notion that I was a pussy man was mostly an idea in my head—until Mali offered me this unexpected opportunity to really delve into what that idea meant to me. Though I'd told Mali how much I loved hers many times before, it became apparent that she hadn't been fully able to take in my appreciation because she didn't yet understand why pussies were beautiful in the first place. They all have their own personality and individuality, their unique curves and coloring. As we explored her pictorial collection, I described to her how each one had its own rare beauty.

When the moment came for me to shift the spotlight and make Mali the center of attention, I was filled with excitement. I gathered up a couple of mirrors and a camera and used them to show her that she was gorgeous from every perspective and that she, too, had a picture-perfect pussy. And later, as I was making love to her, I could sense that she was more receptive to my adoration and touch than she'd ever been before.

For both of us, this experience was profoundly meaningful and revelatory as well as intensely pleasurable. It also felt multidimensional, integrating all the realms of connection—physical, creative, emotional, and spiritual—and culminating in a profound feeling of unity and aliveness. To us, this is sex with genuine soul.

As a couple, the power of developing erotic versatility is that it gives you unlimited sexual potential together. By welcoming your entire selves—bodies, minds, hearts, and souls—into your shared experiences, you have an enormous sexual arena in which to play. And when you're both willing to explore and evolve across all dimensions, that arena will continue to expand and excite you.

In addition, couples who speak of having soulful sexual experiences sometimes mention how their depth of love and connection positively affects not only their own relationship, but all aspects of their lives and the people around them. And they wonder: if more people were creating such joyful experiences for themselves, what kind of effect might that have on the world as a whole?

4

THE PSYCHOLOGY OF PHENOMENAL SEX

Whatever our age, experience, or sexual history, we all have our "stuff" around sex. Practically everyone has suffered from some degree of poor body image or low self-esteem. There may be aspects of our sexuality that we feel embarrassed, nervous, or confused about. And we probably all have thoughts, desires, or experiences we've never shared with anyone out of shame, guilt, or fear.

No matter how we might try to keep our "stuff" to ourselves, if we don't acknowledge and find ways to address these things, they will eventually affect our relationship. You've probably experienced the sometimes-frustrating truth that intimacy has a way of bringing to the surface anything that is unconscious, unacknowledged, or unhealed in us. As you and your partner continue to grow your sexual connection, you'll find that any sex-related fears, resistances, anxieties, or other issues won't stay hidden away for long. Believe it or not, this doesn't have to be a bad thing. Bringing these issues out into the open, where they can be acknowledged, explored, and even healed, can help keep your sexual connection feeling healthy and alive.

When you have an intention to approach anything that could be an *obstacle* to connection as an *opportunity* for connection, every issue that affects you sexually can become a catalyst for deepening intimacy. Two people who have built a solid foundation of safety and trust, and who can be vulnerable and authentic with each other, can make substantial progress in just a weekend together. Dinners and movies can be fun, but helping each other work through a fear or limitation is exhilarating because you're relating on an entirely new level of intimacy.

It's unbelievably rewarding to help the one you love make progress in overcoming a limitation they've struggled with. Just imagine the love and gratitude you would feel for a partner who supported you in making a personal breakthrough and becoming less fearful, more open, or more self-accepting. And lovemaking is even more fulfilling when you become willing to experiment with something you've always avoided or take a leap forward and accept something about yourself you previously couldn't.

In this chapter, we present a variety of techniques for approaching many of the common issues related to sexuality—whether physical, psychological, or emotional—as opportunities for healing, growth, sensuality, and pleasure. We will explore ways that lovers can

- Help one another overcome mental, emotional, or physical barriers to intimacy
- Identify and dispel misperceptions or self-defeating ideas about their bodies or their sexuality
- Uncover and transform feelings of low self-esteem, guilt, shame, or insecurity
- Heal lingering issues stemming from past experiences that were traumatic or felt shameful

Helping each other lessen the effects of or even dissolve issues like these is one of the most intimate experiences two people can share. Recent research into successful long-term relationships confirms that when partners support each other in overcoming personal obstacles and becoming their best selves, their relationship thrives.[1]

By assisting each other in this way, you not only expand your sexual possibilities together, you also inspire feelings of warmth, happiness, and gratitude. And what's not to love about that?

The techniques you'll encounter in the following stories combine elements of psychology with empathy, creativity, and eroticism. Although mental health professionals often suggest techniques like these to their clients, these practical, common-sense approaches existed long before psychologists named, studied, and refined them. Your great-grandmother probably intuitively knew that thinking about something in a different way could make you feel differently about that thing (a skill psychologists call "cognitive reframing") or that gradual, repeated exposure to something that seems scary will increase one's comfort with that thing over time ("immersion therapy"). By adapting these simple tools to the unique situations that arise in your relationship, you can help each other shed limiting beliefs, heal from your pasts, and come into your full sexual potential—together.

Of course, bringing your intimate thoughts, feelings, fears, and desires out into the open requires an environment in which you're at ease with expressing yourselves authentically. Remember to practice the six keys to intimate adventures (see chapter 2) and the two essential elements for emotional connection (empathy and reassurance) to help create a safe, receptive, and supportive space.

Once you see how other people have used these techniques, you'll likely find yourselves thinking about creative ways to approach something that has been preventing the two of you from fully expressing and enjoying yourselves. For example, if there are sexual activities that make one of you uncomfortable, such as having sex in a particular location or position or experimenting with a certain toy, you might dream up ways to make new, positive, and pleasurable associations with those things. Or if one of you is being held back by a lack of self-acceptance, like the belief that some body part is too small or too large, it might be possible to design an erotic experience to help ease those concerns. You'll both begin to see that whenever a limitation or resistance comes up around some aspect of intimacy or sexuality, there just might be a way for it to actually bring you closer together.

This understanding will also serve you well in the future, as time has a way of presenting all of us with new and unexpected challenges. One thing's for sure: your bodies, libidos, and desires *will* change. For the sake of your relationship and your sexual connection, you want to be ready for those changes.

By becoming more comfortable in your bodies and with your desires, you will grow in sexual self-confidence and feel even more connected. And the explorations that get you there will be both pleasurable and memorable.

COGNITIVE REFRAMING: TELLING YOURSELF A BETTER STORY

The idea behind this first technique is that we all view everything that happens to us through our own particular lens or frame. No two people respond to or interpret the same event in exactly the same way. And our interpretation of any event can greatly influence our emotional experience of that event. Cognitive reframing involves identifying, challenging, and then changing or "reframing" negative or unhelpful thoughts and associations. Another way to think about this idea is that we're all continually telling ourselves a story about what's happening in our lives, and telling ourselves a better story can radically change how we're feeling about what's happening.

The ability to look at something from a new and more positive perspective has been proven to make for a happier life and is a skill taught by psychologists, teachers, and parents alike.[2] Rather than just reacting to feelings such as worry or fear, cognitive reframing involves engaging our higher-reasoning skills to question the relevance or validity of the thoughts that produced those feelings. Reframing can also help us overcome "negativity bias," which is the tendency to place more importance on bad experiences than on good or neutral ones.

The basic technique is pretty simple. When a feeling like anxiety or insecurity arises, follow this four-step process:

Step 1. Examine the thoughts that are behind that emotion. If you can't pinpoint exact thoughts, imagine what thoughts *could* have produced the emotion. Working with them will be just as effective.

Step 2. Assess the influence these thoughts have on you. Are they preventing you from feeling confident and comfortable? Are they limiting your ability to feel connected to your partner?

Step 3. Ask yourself how your experience would be different if you were free from these thoughts and the emotional state they induce.

Step 4. Find an alternate perspective—an idea that is just as true as (or truer than) the original idea, and one that will give you a better experience. Shift your focus to that idea instead.

Here's an example of this process in action. Suppose Zina and Sage are making love, having a wonderful time together. Then Zina catches a glimpse of herself in the mirror and instantly starts to feel uncomfortable, embarrassed, and even a little depressed. This feeling of discomfort could be her cue to check in. She might recognize that she was thinking something like, "My stomach is hanging down. That looks so ugly!" She could then ask herself, *Is this thought preventing me from feeling relaxed and connected to Sage?* "Absolutely!" *How would my experience be different if I were free from this thought?* "I'd really be enjoying myself, like I was a few minutes ago." *What's a better idea for me to focus on?* Zina might decide to focus instead on a thought like, "Sage loves me just the way I am and isn't thinking about my stomach." Or, because thoughts themselves can be a barrier to arousal and intimacy, Zina might interrupt her negative thinking altogether by putting her full attention on the sensations in her body.

When you get the hang of this process, you can often alter your mood dramatically in a matter of minutes.

Cognitive reframing is a powerful technique, and one you'll want to practice so it'll be there when you need it. You can use it on your own, as Zina did in the example above. In addition, assisting each other with this on occasion by offering alternative perspectives and interpretations can accelerate the process in an intimate way.

In her previous relationships, fear about how she might look when she was having an orgasm kept Alexis from fully letting go. "I just couldn't allow myself to get out of control and risk making a really strange face," she says. When she started seeing Will, she could tell that holding herself back from expressing her passion was keeping them from being as connected as they could be. So one night she took a chance and confessed her fear to him.

"He immediately reassured me that seeing unbridled passion on a woman's face is the sexiest thing on earth," Alexis says. "He said that when a woman lets herself express what she's feeling, she's beautiful."

Her boyfriend's reassurance helped Alexis begin to let go of her worries about her appearance. Now when she recognizes that she's holding herself back because of what she might look like, Alexis reminds herself of Will's more positive perspective: that the passion and pleasure expressed on her face is sexy and beautiful.

"Not worrying about what I look like," Alexis reports, "sets my orgasms free!" Will says that helping Alexis feel more comfortable with her natural expressions of passion is just as exciting for him. "Watching the woman I love really let go is a super turn-on for me!" he says.

By inviting you to see yourself in another way, as Will did for Alexis, your partner can help you heal limiting or self-defeating beliefs. Of course, you must be open to hearing their ideas, so watch that you don't just outright reject them. Instead, take time to consider whether there's something useful in what they have to say.

Shannon has a habit of comparing herself negatively with other women whenever she and her husband Russell go out. Shannon says that opening up to Russell about this tendency has helped shine light into a dark place. "We talk about the fact that there will always be people cuter, smarter, or wealthier than us anywhere we go, but that I'm beautiful and successful too," she says. "Remembering that truth when I start to get down on myself is really helpful."

Russell has given Shannon the green light to tell him about any self-disparaging thoughts she's having when they're out together. She says, "He might tell me, 'You're right, she's really beautiful. And so are you!' It helps so much to have that quick reassurance from him. Especially when he says something like, 'Don't forget, you've got gorgeous eyes, you have the hottest ass ever, and I'm totally in love with you!'" Repeating Russell's compliments helps settle down her negative self-talk. So if she hears herself thinking, "She's so much more put together than I am," she might giggle to herself, "Yeah, but I have the hottest ass ever!"

Here's one more example of how a little cognitive reframing can make sex much more enjoyable. One Saturday afternoon, sometime during the first few months that Joe and I (Mali) were dating, Joe must have noticed a fleeting look of discomfort or displeasure on my face during an intense lovemaking session. Or maybe he sensed a little holding back on my part. Whatever it was, he stopped what he was doing and sweetly asked me what was up.

It took a little coaxing to get me to confess what was going through my head and taking me out of the moment. But I finally told him, and it was this: I thought my breasts looked a whole lot better when I was lying on my back than when I was on my hands and knees.

With that revelation, Joe gave me a smile, a kiss, and a pep talk I'll never forget.

"When you're lying on your back," he explained, "your breasts are beautiful, very symmetrical, right up against your chest. They look artistic and sensual. When you're on your hands and knees, they become more sexual. They turn into tits. And those tits are very sexy! When they're hanging down, moving in rhythm with our bodies, they become part of our sexual experience. They're in sexual motion!"

I was stunned. This idea of making a distinction between "breasts" and "tits" was revolutionary for me. Here was this sex position that I loved the feel of but had never felt completely comfortable in because I'd always thought it made my breasts look ugly. I'd never talked about it before with anyone. I'd just felt ashamed about it.

With his observation, Joe gave me an entirely new frame through which to view my breasts, one that worked far better than the one I'd used in the past. I've reminded myself of this perspective many times in the years since ("Those are your tits, girl, not your breasts!" I'll say to myself), resulting in me feeling far less inhibited and even more in love with Joe.

Joe's help here was essential to the shift in my self-perception. This was not an alternative perspective I would ever have reached on my own! We've done this type of thing often enough now that we both know that if we can gather the courage to reveal the negative story we've been telling ourselves, the other will be there to help us craft a new and better one.

Once you and your lover discover the power in helping each other rewrite scripts that are holding you back, you'll find yourselves inspired to rewrite as many as possible!

IMMERSION THERAPY: EASING INTO IT

Another versatile healing technique often employed by psychologists, immersion therapy involves gradually introducing someone to an object or situation that causes them fear or anxiety. Whether it's a fear of public speaking, a fear of heights, or a fear of cunnilingus, the basic idea is to create a safe environment to ease the person into the circumstances that bring on their discomfort so they can learn to relax around them. The idea is nothing new. Some version of immersion therapy has probably been around longer than parents have been helping their children get over being afraid of the dark!

So many issues that surface around sexuality could be helped with a lovers' version of immersion therapy. For example, many of us have developed certain resistances or limitations that can affect our ability to be intimate. Some people don't want to be touched in a particular place or way, while others resist hugging or even kissing because they feel awkward or claustrophobic. Other people, because of dissatisfaction with their bodies, will only make love with the lights off or are reluctant to be seen in certain positions. Even if a limitation might not seem like a big deal—such as a resistance to having one's hair touched or to sex in the morning—it can still give the two of you something new to explore sexually. And exploring new sexual territory together makes sex endlessly intriguing!

Here's an example of how this might look. I (Mali) was born with visual defects that rendered me virtually sightless in one eye and with limited vision in the other. Becoming totally blind has always been one of my greatest fears. I've never been turned on by the idea of being blindfolded, despite the fact that this appears on almost every list of suggestions for bringing more excitement into your sex life. So when Joe said he thought it would be sexy to blindfold and then make love to me, it would have been very easy for me to simply say the idea didn't interest me and leave it at that. Joe, being a considerate lover, would have honored my decision. But I recognized that my resistance meant this was a sexual edge for me—and that meant it was also a sexual opportunity.

Exploring that uncomfortable edge with Joe, it wasn't long before I realized there was more to my resistance than a fear of sightlessness. It was also related to a deeply rooted fear of being attacked or violated. We talked about my trepidations, and Joe did everything he could to make me feel safe and at ease. First, he had me tie on the blindfold myself, a simple scarf that I could easily remove at any moment. He put on music I love, which also helped me relax. Then he began to stroke my body from my face down to my toes. As he caressed me, creating delicious sensations throughout my body, he spoke softly to me, reassuring me that I was safe and that nothing would harm me. He had me take slow, deep breaths to help me let go of any tension I was feeling. All of this allowed me to slowly immerse myself in the experience of being blindfolded for a while.

I've always been a "lights on" girl, and yet, with Joe's encouragement, I've discovered that sex in the dark has its advantages too. Taking away any one sense heightens all the others. Without vision, I was very aware of Joe's movements, the sound of his breathing, the warmth emanating from his body. And his touch felt electric! Each time we've tried this since, it takes time for him to help me relax, and that is a fun part of the process.

From my (Joe's) perspective, alongside the excitement of doing something unusual together, helping Mali overcome this limitation has been really rewarding. I'm also aware that when she's blindfolded, I have to be especially sensitive and really tuned in to her. I have to say, being able to calm her down when she's feeling nervous, and help her be receptive to my love and attention, is a useful skill both in and out of the bedroom.

Let's look at a few more examples of people who instinctively used a process of gradual immersion to help their lover let go of a resistance, fear, or anxiety.

The first time her new love mentioned the name of a former girlfriend, Janelle totally shut down. Lyle noticed immediately. "What's coming up for you?" he asked gently. "It's as though you're not even here with me."

When Janelle came out of her dark place and shared with Lyle that she couldn't bear hearing about his ex-girlfriends, that it made her terribly upset, Lyle told her, "I don't ever want you to have to close yourself off to me like that. Whatever it is that's making you feel this way, I know we can find our way through it—together. I'm here for you, no matter what!"

This loving gesture changed everything. It created a safe place for Janelle to reveal to Lyle the origins of her sensitivity. She'd been married for ten years to a frequently jealous and angry man who insisted that neither of them ever say the name of a former partner aloud. Now, because Lyle made Janelle feel safe and understood, they were actually able to begin reminiscing together, a little at a time, about their past relationships.

Lyle told Janelle about his very first love, a girl he met the summer he was eight. The romance was so innocent that Janelle found herself connecting with Lyle as a sweet, loving boy. Over time, as they shared more of their stories, Janelle came to understand that she really was safe with Lyle and that he would never react with jealousy or anger if she mentioned a previous partner. Janelle describes this very personal experience with immersion therapy as a "slow, loving healing process."

Here's another example. On a couple of occasions, Sandra had let her husband know that she'd love to watch him masturbate. The first time she asked, Rob said he didn't feel like it. The second time, he admitted he just wasn't comfortable with the idea. Sandra told Rob she understood and would just enjoy her vision in fantasy, but that if he ever changed his mind, she'd be thrilled.

Sandra's accepting attitude made it possible for Rob to eventually open up about the reason for his reluctance: his mother had barged into his room when he was a teenager and caught him "playing Uno." After telling him he'd "go to hell for all eternity," she punished him.

Sandra's understanding and loving response to his admission

made Rob willing to try an experiment. On his next trip out of town, he would try masturbating while they had an audio-only phone-sex date. Being on the phone created safety for Rob, as he didn't have to worry about actually being seen. This was an exciting experience for them both—so much so that he suggested they try it again the next night. With Sandra's reassurance that these sessions were wickedly hot, Rob came home ready to take their new adventure from the phone into the flesh.

By now, you're probably starting to see a pattern in the qualities present in these interactions. In each instance, the partner offered their support from a place of acceptance and without expectations. And the person with the sensitivity had complete control over how, and even if, that sensitivity was explored. Look for these crucial elements in the stories that follow about two more couples.

As a child, Priya had been molested by an uncle who performed oral sex on her over a period of years. Although she had seen a therapist in her twenties and felt she had worked through much of the trauma and pain of those childhood experiences, Priya had never been able to tolerate cunnilingus. To protect herself, she instinctively tightened up whenever someone she was seeing attempted to go down on her. Sometime in her early forties, however, Priya started wishing she could finally let go of this fear.

Then Priya met Adrian, a sensitive and loving man with whom she soon felt safe enough to reveal this traumatic part of her past, as well as her desire to one day actually enjoy receiving oral sex. Adrian said he would be honored to explore Priya's desire with her. He assured her they could move very slowly and would never go beyond what she was ready for.

Initially, Priya would lay back on the bed, sometimes clothed, sometimes in just her underwear. Adrian would simply kiss and caress her body while she focused on relaxing. Over time, as she felt more at ease and invited him to move closer, he was able to kiss all along the edges of her panties without her becoming tense. Eventually, Adrian was able to kiss on top of them, lightly at first and then with more pressure. Whenever Priya felt any anxiety starting up, she would say so and Adrian would immediately back off—not only until she was fully relaxed again, but until she explicitly urged him to continue.

Priya says she understands now that although the years she spent in therapy were essential for her healing process, her eventual comfort with oral sex had to happen "in the arms of a patient and understanding man."

As far back as she can remember, Cassidy had been attracted to the idea of being tied up and "taken." But she'd also felt very conflicted about this desire, as just the thought of it actually happening filled her with panic. Two years into her relationship with Nick, Cassidy felt so close to him that she divulged her desire to be restrained by a lover, as well as the inner conflict she experienced at the actual prospect. Nick was quite excited to be able to help Cassidy explore this desire.

After talking about some things they might try, they agreed to begin with Nick gently holding Cassidy's hands behind her back while he kissed her. "Even that was pretty intense," she says. They talked about the fears that were coming up for her. Nick reminded her to breathe, reassuring her that she was in a safe place, that no one was going to hurt her, and that they could stop at any time.

As their experiments slowly intensified, Nick learned to sense when Cassidy started to tense up, as well as how he could use "a combination of logic and love" to help her quiet her fears. Eventually she trusted that he would never push her too far, and she was able to completely relax and enjoy being restrained and "taken" by the man she loves and trusts.

Laying the Foundation and Creating Safety

So many of us who feel uncertain, insecure, or fearful around some aspect of sexuality could benefit from a gradual introduction to, and greater relaxation around, that discomfort or anxiety. A safe, loving environment and a willing, creative partner are what made it possible for each of the people in these stories to face and begin to let go of their negative feelings and associations and form new, more positive ones.

If you have an opportunity to try a similar approach to something that's holding you or your lover back in some way, the following guidelines will help ensure that your experiences are both positive and healing:

- **Connection comes first.** Yes, you've heard that before. We can't stress enough that it's a strong emotional connection and deep sense of real trust that give a couple the necessary foundation from which to create such life-changing experiences together. So make your connection your priority, rather than any particular progress or result. Never sacrifice your connection by trying to rush the process of helping your partner move past a fear or limitation—or, if you're the one being helped, by putting pressure on yourself to please your partner. If you're feeling the need to speed things up, that's precisely when slowing down and offering extra servings of loving reassurance can make a world of difference.
- **Being heard is healing.** Just sharing our feelings of shame or embarrassment with someone we trust can be tremendously healing and freeing. If your partner is open to a conversation about a fear or limitation, you might ask what in particular they find unpleasant or irritating or scary, how contemplating that makes them feel, and where their resistance might stem from. If together you decide to try a particular approach, keep checking in about any

fears or negative thoughts they might be having during the experience. Reassure them that they're in a safe, supportive place. It's highly unlikely that they will be healed from their fear or limitation all at once (although that can happen), so make this an ongoing conversation, an open door for sharing any new thoughts, ideas, or observations either of you has.

- **Seek support.** Whatever the issue is, others have been through it and help is available. Educate yourselves by reading books or articles on the topic together. Involving a counselor can often be beneficial, particularly if you can't think of ways to approach the issue or if you make some progress but then feel stuck. If the fear or anxiety is related to trauma or abuse, or is particularly deep or intense, consulting someone who specializes in that field can be invaluable.

- **Get creative.** Do you remember that creative dimension of sexual connection? This is where it comes in very handy! Together, imagine some small steps the two of you might take to explore the issue you've identified. Your partner may land on an idea or two by contemplating the following questions: *If I were to have moved beyond this issue one day, what would it have taken to get me there? What experiences would I have had?*

- **Check your agenda at the door.** People often feel embarrassed, guarded, or defensive around sexual issues and limitations, so a "no judgment, no pressure" atmosphere is essential. If the two of you decide to try one of the ideas you've come up with, make sure that neither of you has a timeline or agenda for your lover's progress. Reassure your partner that they're in charge of how fast and how far any exploration goes and that you're committed to supporting them no matter what. Over time, your lover will come to know that they really can trust you with their insecurities—and their transformations.

- **Stay at the edge of their comfort zone.** As you explore your partner's edge with them, do your best never to push them beyond it. As they eventually realize that they're safe here and can actually begin to relax, their comfort zone will expand naturally.

With a lighthearted, loving attitude and an intention to feel connected all the way through, you'll be creating experiences that are both profoundly intimate and profoundly healing.

What Would You Do?

Let's look at a few hypothetical situations in which a gradual exposure to the source of someone's discomfort, while helping them feel safe and relaxed, could enable them to grow more at ease. Although every person and every relationship is unique, we've offered some possible approaches for each scenario to inspire you to think creatively about how *you* might help a lover in similar circumstances.

Suppose you're with someone who doesn't like to be touched in a certain place, such as their feet, ears, or face. If they're open to a conversation, you might learn something about where their aversion comes from. The source could be emotional, such as someone who doesn't like their face touched because they think their face is unattractive. If they're receptive to it, you might ask them to imagine what it would feel like to have their face touched by someone who loves it (you!). Or offer them an everything-but-the-face massage: stroke their shoulders, neck, ears, and hair, while they focus on accepting and enjoying your loving attention. Eventually, if you turn the lights low, close your eyes, or even wear a blindfold, they may relax enough to lie with their head in your lap while you caress their face. Set aside any expectations about the outcome of your explorations. While it might happen in an afternoon, it could take much longer for a person to fully believe that *you* believe their face is lovable and touchable.

An aversion like this can also be the result of a bad experience or physical discomfort. Maurice, for example, doesn't like anyone touching his hair because of the nerve damage he sustained in a serious car accident. In a situation like this, someone may have no interest in exploring their limitation because change may not be possible or would take more energy than it's worth.

Now imagine that your lover doesn't like to French kiss. Through a conversation, you learn about the time that a blind date wrapped his hands tightly around their neck and attempted to force his tongue down their throat. Any kissing that involves the tongue brings back that traumatic memory. If they're open to exploring this edge with you, you might describe what *you* love about this type of sensual kissing, such as the intimate way it feels or how it can be slow and gentle and involve sweet touches and caresses. Your description could be just the enticement they need to give it a try with you. Or you might suggest a hot make-out session with no mouth-to-mouth contact, using your lips and tongues to explore each other's shoulders, ears, face, and neck. Or kiss passionately, but only using your lips. In any of these explorations, your lover is always in charge—any tongue play will be theirs. A few safe and sensuous kissing sessions, indulging in all the ways your lips can dance together, and your lover may feel the building of desire for a little "French" after all.

Notice again how important it is that the person with the sensitivity be given unconditional and complete control of the situation. They need reassurance that there are no expectations and that it's absolutely okay for them to decide, at any moment, not to take the exploration any further.

Now suppose the person you're with doesn't like to hug because they find it claustrophobic. Hugs are easy to make gradual progress with, as they are simple to engage in and simple to let go of and can happen in a variety of settings. If they're up for a little experimenting, you could try a playful faux hug, wrapping your arms around each other without allowing your bodies to actually touch. Walk arm-in-arm—essentially a sideways hug—or embrace them from behind (with their consent) while you watch some live music or a sunset together. Gently draw them out about how these interactions make them feel, and experiment with just how lightly you have to be touching for their feelings of claustrophobia to quiet down. If they're eventually willing to try a longer hug, let them guide it, reassuring them that they can let go at any point. To give them something positive to focus on, you might describe what you love about hugging, such as feeling your physical or emotional connection, your hearts beating together, or your shared warmth.

Imagine your lover tells you their nipples are just too sensitive to be touched or played with. Like other physical sensitivities, nipple sensitivity can be a reaction to a traumatic experience, a side effect of a medication or medical condition, or have no apparent cause at all. Let's say your lover reveals that when she was a girl, the neighbor boys were obsessed with "tittie twisters" and would frequently grab and wrench her nipples until it brought tears to her eyes. To this day, she associates having her nipples touched with pain, humiliation, and unwanted sexual contact.

With empathy and reassurance, you might be able to create a zone of safety in which some healing around this can take place. Let her know you'll do your best never to touch her nipples unless and until she invites you to. Enjoy touching and caressing her breasts in every way you can while keeping your promise, and assure her that it's actually erotic for you to lust after her nipples and *not* be able to play with them.

Someday, if she feels ready, you can talk about what might allow her to relax while her nipples receive some kind of loving attention. If she's willing, you can try laying your palm against her chest, perhaps over her clothing, letting her feel the weight of your hand but without any potentially distracting or irritating motion. Or press your tongue flat over her nipple, again remaining motionless, to see if she can get comfortable with that gentle pressure. If she's able to enjoy touch like this and welcomes further exploration, try it many times so that she can fully trust that you won't move beyond what she's ready for. If she can touch her own nipples in a way that feels good to her, she might take your fingers or hands and guide them to move in the same way. Throughout all of this, keep talking about any uncomfortable thoughts or emotions that come up for her, and help her to calm them by reminding her that she is safe, loved, and completely in charge.

Let's examine one more hypothetical scenario. Suppose you're with someone who doesn't enjoy giving or receiving oral sex (or both). There could be many possible and understandable reasons behind such a dislike. Some people are reluctant to be the recipient because the sensations are too intense or, conversely, not stimulating at all. Others might feel too vulnerable, perhaps as the result of experiences with previous sex partners who went straight for the most sensitive areas without warming them up first or who were too rough or aggressive. For some women, an aversion to performing fellatio might be related to seeing porn of women being forced against their will or obviously not enjoying what they're doing or to having been with men who tried to act out such aggressive or abusive scenes without their consent.

Talking about the origins of your partner's reluctance, if they can identify them, will help you explore this opportunity together. For example, if they fear you going down on them because they're so sensitive, they could show you exactly where a little attention might actually feel good, and describe precisely the degree and kind of attention they're imagining. You, of course, won't move beyond those boundaries until they ask you to (or beg you to!). Or you might carefully and methodically explore the entire area together, experimenting with different kinds of touch and pressure. If at any point they tighten up in self-protection, back off until they're relaxed again.

If your partner has never liked giving oral sex but is interested in learning how to enjoy it, they can try a little oral foreplay now and then—just adding in a bit of kissing, licking, or gentle sucking around your genital area while you're making love. Sustaining eye contact can help some people feel more connected during oral-genital play. If your partner can't seem to let go of a fear of being hurt while they're going down on you, you might suggest they bind your wrists and ankles to a chair and take total control!

Exploring at the edges of your sexual comfort zones might just become your go-to approach for any resistance, fear, or limitation either of you uncovers in yourselves. By viewing your own limitations as opportunities, you may well discover that they are one of your most direct paths to deepening your intimacy and strengthening your connection with your beloved partner.

MINDFUL SEXUALITY: CULTIVATING AWARENESS AND CURIOSITY

One of the greatest areas of growth in psychology today is the use of mindfulness. Especially helpful for reducing stress and anxiety, mindful-based approaches have found popularity with everyone from mothers to managers to millionaires. Learning how to quiet our busy minds is more necessary than ever in this world of distractions and multitasking. We rarely allow ourselves the luxury of doing just one thing at a time. Mindful practices, which include breathing and meditation exercises, can help us feel more relaxed, more present in our bodies, and more connected to the world around us.

Psychologist and sex researcher Lori A. Brotto has conducted extensive research into the use of mindfulness for treating issues related to libido, arousal, and orgasm in women.[3] Her findings overwhelmingly show that mindful-awareness practices can significantly improve sexual desire and satisfaction. Mindfulness is also proving to be helpful for premature ejaculation and difficulties attaining or maintaining an erection.

At its heart, being mindful is simply giving your full attention to whatever you're doing right now. By noticing when your attention is being distracted by something else, you can gently steer it back to this moment. To put it simply, if you want sex to be more exciting and fulfilling, *be there* while it's happening instead of mentally being somewhere else.

Linda and Paul: The Mindful Path to Pleasure

Linda and Paul, a couple in their fifties who started dating after both being single for several years, discovered for themselves the link between mindfulness and sexual satisfaction. Prior to their meeting, Linda had been diagnosed with vaginal atrophy, a very common condition that makes intercourse difficult and painful. Linda's atrophy was severe and possibly the result of many years of sexual inactivity combined with the effects of menopause.

"For years I thought well, I'm going to spend the rest of my life alone, because a sexual relationship just isn't possible for me. But eventually the loneliness got so extreme that I knew I was just going to have to allow myself to be vulnerable and see what happened. I also knew I needed to find somebody who would accept this about me. It was scary, but if I didn't try, I would never know."

From the moment they met, Linda and Paul loved being in each other's company, and they started spending more and more time together. Before she even got up the courage to talk about her condition and the possibility that she might never be able to have vaginal intercourse, Paul eased her mind. "I was so anxious and scared, and he said, 'We don't have to do anything we don't feel comfortable doing. Let's just feel good.' His words put me at ease, and we were able to talk about not only my condition but concerns Paul had as well."

Linda wasn't the only one who hadn't been intimate with anyone for a long time. Paul was anxious too, yet very much wanted a loving relationship. He wanted Linda to know that intercourse wasn't that important to him in a relationship—but sharing sexual feelings together was. "There's a whole lot we can do without having intercourse!" he assured her.

In order to be sexually intimate, Linda says, they had to break free of the common perception that sex equals intercourse. "What do we do with this desire, this sexual energy we're feeling? How are we going to express it when the only way we know isn't available to us?" they asked themselves. "If we can't have traditional intercourse, what is our sex life?"

To answer these questions, Linda says, "We had to let ourselves explore and be open to whatever the other person needed to feel sexy, to feel arousal, to feel pleasure. We had to know that whatever that is, is perfectly okay, and good." This, Linda explains, "is where the mindfulness comes in. Cluing into what the other person is responding to requires your total focus. You have to pay attention to their breathing, their muscular tensions and releases, and any sounds or verbalizations they're making, and connect that to what you're doing: your pressure, your tempo."

What Linda is describing may sound obvious, but all too often, people are not fully aware of the connection between what they're doing and how their lover is responding. This awareness, Linda says, took time, attention, and patience to acquire. "We had to start by focusing on one of us at a time, and sometimes guiding each other, their hands or their mouth." It wasn't until several months into their relationship, she says, "after developing this rhythm together, that we could pay attention to the other person and not lose awareness of our own sensations of pleasure." Paul adds, "We learned that focusing on giving the other person pleasure increased our own pleasure."

For Linda, mindful sexuality involves "suspending all judgment, both of your partner and of yourself. I also had to stop thinking that what we were doing was not really sex and open my mind to a new concept of sex. When we got together, we let go of any preconceived notions of what sex is and followed our instincts about what felt good, sexy, and loving. It's totally different for us than I ever experienced before, or imagined it could be, or even imagined I would be okay with. And it's much more satisfying than either one of us has experienced before."

Being mindful also means quieting the mental chatter. "For me, everything about sex used to be a thought. I was always overthinking and overanalyzing. Even though I'm a very verbal person, I'm learning not to put a label on the moment, to just pay attention."

Through these practices, Linda has developed much more awareness of what her body is feeling at any moment. "To become aware of when you're aroused is a big deal!" she says. "I now recognize that Paul's touch giving me a little tingle is the beginning of being aroused. It's my body's response to him. I can ignore that tingling, or I can notice it and let it blossom."

Linda has also learned to pay attention to when something is too much. If we can't acknowledge or communicate when we're not feeling good, we will start to pull back, shut down, or go numb. "We're able to say to each other, 'I'm feeling overstimulated and need to back off.' He's actually better at this than I am," she laughs.

Like meditation, mindfulness takes intention. "Every time we're together requires that commitment to being mindful," Linda says. "Even simple things like turning on mood music or adjusting the lights or temperature in the room can be a part of intentionally letting the other person know that you're ready and willing to be with them 100 percent."

Linda and Paul want people to know that the intimacies of sex without intercourse can be completely fulfilling. "There are so many people struggling with similar issues who are afraid to even go online and meet someone. That's why I was single for ten years," Linda says. "People who think they have to have intercourse to have sex have no idea how powerful the alternatives can be in finding intimacy with each other. Our sex life is just as, if not more, intimate than any intercourse either of us had before we met. I'm not sure Paul and I would have developed the intimacy we share now without having had to learn new ways to express our sexual passion for each other."

Paul expresses what they've discovered together this way: "What we have is all love. Just love. Sex isn't a separate thing."

"He taught me that. It's how he got me into bed in the first place!" Linda laughs. "I went into this whole dating thing expecting that I would find a companion, someone I could do things with and go out to dinner with, so that I wouldn't be as lonely. I didn't expect this!"

A Field Guide for Mindful Lovemaking

In addition to clearing out distractions (like tucking the kids into bed and putting the phones away) and making sure the room is clean, warm, and smells good (try lighting a candle or burning some essential oil), here are a few other ways to bring more mindfulness to your lovemaking:

- **Free your mind of to-dos.** If there are tasks on your mind that you have to remember, like a call you need to make tomorrow, clear them from your headspace by writing yourself a note or setting a reminder. By assuring they won't be forgotten, you release the burden of trying to remember them or feeling anxious about them. We even believe it's okay to jot something down even in the heat of the moment so that it doesn't continue to be a mental distraction. Some people will say that pausing a sex session for the sake of a to-do list will take you out of the moment, but a few seconds' pause is far better than struggling for the next hour to stop thinking about something while simultaneously trying to make sure you don't forget it!

- **Expect not, want not.** Anytime you have a picture of what sex will or should look like, you limit spontaneity and the possibility for something new or unexpected to happen. You might waste time and energy trying to make what's happening align with that image and feel worried or frustrated if it doesn't. In the midst of that, you certainly won't be able to fully enjoy whatever *is* happening! By having a minimum of expectations, you can come to each other with openness and receptivity and let a brand new experience unfold. Mantras, or simple statements you silently repeat to yourself, may sound silly, but you might be surprised at how a little mental reminder like, "Everything is okay here" can make it easier for you to relax and bring your full attention back to what you're doing. Or try "There's nowhere else I have to be, nothing else I have to do" or "This feels good. I feel good."
- **Get skin to skin.** It's hard to get in the mood if you're feeling stressed or anxious or have physical tension or pain. A few minutes of massaging each other can help ease tense muscles as well as mental distractions. From there, you can move to some sensual touch, exploring each other's bodies with no intention to stimulate or turn on. Just enjoy the physicality of flesh against flesh[4] and all the sensations being evoked in you. You might also express what types of touch are arousing to you, without either of you having to act on that arousal. As always, if anything feels uncomfortable, you might have just discovered another opportunity for intimacy.
- **Slow it down. Way down.** Allow yourselves time to sink into being together. Gaze into each other's eyes while letting your thoughts grow quiet. Feel each other's presence. Melt into a long hug while

relaxing any places you're holding tension. Savor a long, slow, sensual kiss. Remind yourselves that the time you have together is precious.

- **Indulge your senses.** If you notice your mind starting to wander—worrying about how you look or that your body isn't responding how you want it to—remember the simple practice of returning your attention to your senses: *What am I feeling, hearing, tasting, smelling, seeing right now?* And when what you're feeling makes you want to moan, squirm, shiver, or sigh, by all means express yourself fully and freely!

- **Bring each other back.** Give your partner permission to call you back to the moment if they sense that your mind might be wandering. They could suggest, for example, that for the next couple of minutes, you put all of your attention on the feeling of their hands moving over your skin. You might even ask for their assistance directly: "I keep thinking about my meeting tomorrow. Help!" By bringing your full awareness back to what's happening right now, you'll be sure to get the most experience out of your experience.

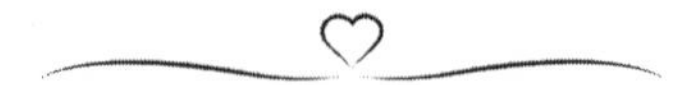

We hope the stories in this chapter have demonstrated that sexual intimacy comes in many forms, each with the ability to be meaningful and pleasurable, and that there are endless ways for couples to work together to overcome hang-ups and insecurities about intimacy. Now let's dive even more deeply into how partners can apply the power of their love and desire to bring about healing, while deepening their bond in the process.

5

THE HEALING POWER OF EROTICISM: WHERE SEX AND LOVE MEET

One special night every fall when I (Mali) was a young girl, I would take my place cross-legged on the floor at my father's feet. My dad would settle back into his recliner, cocktail in hand, eager for the entertainment to come. The annual Miss America pageant was finally here.

As the women glided across the stage, every one of them impossibly elegant and beautiful, my father issued a running commentary on their bodies. Here was a parade of perfect representations of female beauty, and he had something critical to say about every one. Unless, that is, she were well-endowed. Only my father would never say a woman was well-endowed. He'd say, "Get a load of *those* boobs!" If a woman had huge boobs, everything else—her talents, her achievements, or what she might have to say—was irrelevant. The woman with the biggest boobs should win. Obviously.

"It's between Miss Alabama and Miss Wisconsin this year!" he'd triumphantly announce.

My dad's fixation extended well beyond our living room. When we were out at a restaurant, my brothers and I would cringe at the way our father would interact with whoever was unlucky enough to wait on us.

"Geesh, look at the jugs on *her*," he'd mock-whisper to us as she approached.

"How are the steaks tonight, darling?" he would ask, directing the question to her chest.

"They're great. They're thick and juicy."

A grin would spread across his face. "Looks like everything around here is thick and juicy!" he'd snicker, pounding his fist on the table and looking very pleased with himself.

Given my father's obsession with large breasts, and the "bigger is better" culture in which I grew up, it's no surprise that even after I began developing into a woman, I always felt insufficient. Being a sexy, desirable woman, I believed, was simply unattainable for small-chested me. As painful as this was for me at times, if it weren't for my negative belief, I would have missed out on one of the most intimate, exhilarating, and transformational experiences of my life.

Several years after we met, Joe and I had the good fortune to sequester ourselves during a tropical five-day working vacation to put the finishing touches on what would eventually become the "Playing Leapfrog" chapter of our first book. The basic concept was simple but profound: that in a strong, solid relationship, partners can be catalysts for each other's growth and evolution. They can help each other make "leaps" in consciousness: letting go of limiting beliefs, overcoming perceived limitations, and healing from the past. In particular, we were writing about playing leapfrog in the bedroom: helping a lover break through negative beliefs about their bodies and their sexuality, even if those beliefs are long-standing. Immersed as we were in these ideas, it was natural to try them out with the insecurity and embarrassment I still carried about the size of my breasts.

Joe had heard these and similar stories from my childhood. He had reassured me on many occasions that my body was beautiful and more than "enough" for him. Yet somehow his loving words and reassurances weren't quite sufficient to completely cure me of my conviction that I was inherently inadequate.

What began as an afternoon's pursuit stretched out well into the evening. Joe was unwavering in his intention to get me to see that my beliefs about what makes breasts attractive were just that: beliefs. And beliefs, as we proved to ourselves once again that unforgettable day, can definitely be changed.

"We're here today to love and appreciate your breasts," he told me. "No more comparisons. No one else's breasts are important here. No one else's ideas about what is or is not attractive matter here."

I relaxed back against his chest as he wrapped me in his arms. He held my breasts in his hands and spoke soothingly to me. "Any breasts can be sexy," he said, "when they belong to a person who feels sexy inside."

He squeezed me lovingly in his hands.

"These breasts are sexy," he affirmed. "They're a part of you, an extension of your inner sexiness. Whether or not they measure up to what some people think they should look like, *they are sexy*."

We lay together that way for a long time. His sincerity, and the deep sense of caring and trust we had cultivated between us, enabled me to take in everything he was saying as one possible truth.

"As I hold your breasts in my hands, I want you to feel through my touch how much I love and desire them. I'd like you to let go of the idea that they should be any different than they are."

Eventually, once my mental objections had quieted down and I could really feel his love for my breasts, he took my hand and led me into the spacious walk-in shower. As I stood naked under that soothing stream, he talked about how beautiful it was to watch the water flowing over my chest. He even brought a mirror into the shower so we could see the sensual show together. I was captivated. *This* is what he sees when he looks at me? No wonder he loves them!

At some point, Joe suggested I close my eyes and put my attention on the feeling of the warm spray against my naked skin. The sensations were delicious. He had me slowly run my own hands over my breasts. I was amazed by how soft they felt, how sensuous. How could I have never noticed this before?

After our sweet time in the shower, Joe toweled me dry and massaged oil into my skin, reminding me to fully take in his love and desire for me. Then he escorted me back to the bedroom and had me get comfortable.

"If we're rejecting a part of ourselves, our experiences will never be as pleasurable as they could be," he wisely pointed out. He said I'd probably always held myself back from accepting the love and attention my breasts had been offered. This was true. Because I'd believed that my previous lovers couldn't actually be enjoying them, I'd always tried to get the focus off my chest.

I watched as Joe wandered around the condo gathering up a selection of random items—some seashells from the table, fresh flowers, a glass of ice cubes, an assortment of kitchen gadgets—and placed them on the nightstand next to the bed.

"You may not even know what kinds of touch your breasts like," he said quietly as he picked up a chopstick from his collection and began using it to "draw" small circles on my chest. For the next little while, he amused himself with discovering just what would cause me to squirm, giggle, moan, or arch my back in pleasure. All the while, he reassured me that he was very much enjoying himself and encouraged me to relax and surrender to the sensations he was creating in and around my breasts.

"What are you feeling?" he would ask, smiling. "What's it like to have this loving attention on a part of your body that you've rejected for so long?"

I had to admit that I was having the time of my life. All this love and attention was as exhilarating as it was freeing.

He devoted some special time to my nipples, which are, I learned that day, one of his favorite things. It's erotic and exciting, he said, to see and feel my nipples physically respond to him. He experimented with what kinds of touch would coax them into becoming erect, and talked about how he loved watching them change in color as they swelled and relaxed. It's true what he says—nipples are amazing!

After making love to my breasts for literally hours, Joe settled in as I modeled everything I'd brought with me: tops and dresses, bras and bikinis. In our private beauty pageant, there was nothing that was not perfect and nothing that was not perfectly lovable. I felt no fear that I would be negatively judged, no sense of shame or insufficiency. The idea that my breasts were "not enough" was incomprehensible to me now.

In the many years since that extraordinary day, not once have I thought of my breasts as inadequate. Not once. Through his loving attention and determination, Joe had given me a new and lasting positive self-image—one that includes what he delightfully calls my "FPTs." (Okay, here's a hint. The P is for "perfect.") He accomplished this by treating me to a profoundly positive and highly erotic experience of my breasts. In essence, he eroticized them.

The word *erotic*, which means "arousing sexual desire," is derived from the Greek word *erotikós*, "caused by love." This union of sex and love is what makes the process of eroticizing a healing experience. By making something erotic, or "arousing sexual desire," we can help free our partner from what's been preventing them from experiencing greater love, connection, intimacy, and pleasure.

In his brilliant book *The Erotic Mind: Unlocking the Inner Sources of Sexual Passion and Fulfillment*, sex therapist Jack Morin defines eroticism as "the interplay of sexual arousal with the challenges of living and loving." Eroticism, he says, is "the process through which sex becomes meaningful."[1]

The examples that follow illustrate various ways that people in healthy, loving relationships can creatively apply the healing power of eroticism to many common "challenges of living and loving." Even if you never face these exact situations, chances are good that one day you'll have the opportunity to try out a similar approach—and discover for yourselves that helping each other open up to more love and pleasure brings more and deeper meaning into your sexual connection.

EROTICIZING NEGATIVE SELF-PERCEPTIONS

You're probably already aware of how common it is for someone to be more accepting and appreciative of their lover's body than their lover is themselves. If so, you'll appreciate the following ideas for using eroticism to help someone quiet their self-critical voice around some perceived flaw or shortcoming. Not only do such profound experiences produce tremendous love and gratitude, it's also an amazing feeling to help someone you care about make progress toward accepting and possibly even appreciating an aspect of themselves that they've been rejecting.

As you think about how you might apply some of these approaches to your own relationship, remember to keep it light. Just think of them as sexy games you might play or new ways to have a fun and connecting time together.

See What I See

If your lover has a negative perception of some aspect of their appearance while your perspective is more positive, here's a way to shift them into seeing what you're seeing. Ask them to set aside their self-critical thoughts for a short time, say five or ten minutes, and to listen as you describe what *you* see. Their task is to take in your words as your truth. Your viewpoint is just as valid (if not more so!) than theirs, and for this brief period, they are not to resist or reject it, but to accept it as legitimate. Seeing themselves through your eyes, even if only for moments at a time, can give them a new, more positive self-perception.

For example, if your lover sees his own face as unattractive, try this little experiment. Invite him to look in a mirror with you and do his best to turn off the self-defeating tape that's been playing in his head for decades and instead concentrate on listening to and acknowledging *your* truth. Point out and describe what you like about his face: his receptive eyes, their beautiful color, his strong jaw line, his nice teeth. When he's able to see what you're seeing, suggest he try training himself to start noticing those things when he looks at his reflection instead of the things he's conditioned himself to focus on over the years.

Because repetition helps us rewire negative habits, you'll want to repeat this exercise from time to time. It might be especially welcome, for example, before he has to give a presentation or when the two of you are getting dressed for a social event.

Turn It into Art

Sometimes we've been scrutinizing photos of ourselves through our "I'm insufficient" filter for so long that we can be blind to seeing anything positive in them. And yet, with the help of a loving partner, photography offers a way to view ourselves from new, more positive perspectives.

When your partner sees something they like, they can take a few pictures from that angle, and then share what they love about them with you. You focus on momentarily suspending your self-criticism and doing your best to see what they're seeing.

If neither of you is all that skillful with a camera, there are plenty of easy-to-follow online tutorials to help you take better pictures, including tips on lighting, angles, cropping, and editing. Together you can find ways, for example, to photograph the sensual curve of a hip or thigh or the artistic silhouette of a breast or belly. Don't be discouraged if your first shots aren't great. Like any photographer, you may have to take quite a few to get one you both really like.

If your partner loves a particular image of you but you're having trouble seeing it positively, pretend it's someone else you're looking at. We tend to be much less critical of others than we are of ourselves. You might frame one of your favorites as a reminder that you *can* see a photo of yourself as attractive. Many people have also found that a boudoir or lingerie photo shoot with a professional who knows how to put them at ease and photograph them in their best light can have a positive and lasting effect on their self-image.

Find a Role Model

If there's an aspect of themselves that your partner struggles with, help them identify an actor, model, or musician they find attractive who has that body type or feature too. There are also many body-positive activists and role models on social media who demonstrate that "healthy and beautiful" comes in endless forms.

When Alicia started dating Jeff, he frequently mentioned how much he adored her body, but she just couldn't believe he was as enamored as he claimed to be. One evening he pulled out some of his art history textbooks from college. As they turned the pages, he pointed out the features of nude Renaissance masterpieces that reminded him of her. Having these classic role models helped Alicia begin to appreciate her own body as a work of art. On another occasion, she and Jeff talked about the fact that throughout history, different kinds of bodies have been revered as ideal. "So the concept of what's the 'right' or 'best' body type is entirely arbitrary!" Alicia now says.

Have Them Own It

If your partner feels insecure about how they look, remind them that research in neuroscience strongly suggests that rehearsing a new way of feeling about yourself can, over time, actually help you to feel that way. When it's just the two of you, encourage your lover to walk, dance, or move about like they know how handsome or irresistible they are. Reassure them that there's only an audience of one here—and that audience adores them. Your lover may be surprised to discover that projecting a little confidence will not only make them feel more self-assured, but will make you even more attracted to them than you were already!

Make It the Object of Your Desire

If there's an aspect of your partner's body that they're critical of but you're just fine with, ask them to indulge you in allowing that part to be the object of your desire. You might put on some music they enjoy and say something like, "I want you to just focus on the truth that your ass is entirely sexy and beautiful to me." Again, the idea is to entice them to momentarily suspend what they think and take in your perspective instead. Invite them to do anything they'd like to show it off for you: dance, caress it, squeeze it, shake it, whatever they're up for.

Your enthusiastic appreciation is evidence that will counter their negative belief about themselves. You might even ask, "How can this part of you be insufficient if I'm getting this turned on just watching you?" If they're eventually able to relax into this and you're both excited to take this exploration a step further, you might even pleasure yourself while continuing to focus your full erotic attention on that aspect of their body.

An intimate experience like this can bring about a substantial, long-lasting shift in self-acceptance. Your partner will be immensely grateful for your loving assistance, and you will feel gratified for being able to help them in this intimate way. And if they need an occasional booster shot of love and desire, you'll no doubt be happy to oblige!

Make Love to It

Any under-appreciated area of your partner's body can become the focus of your lovemaking for a while. Make love to that area while your partner does their best to let go of their negative thoughts and make a connection with the pleasure you're providing.

Help them get comfortable, perhaps propped up with pillows. A glass of wine and turning the lights down might help too. Candlelight is not only a romantic mood-setter; the light it casts can also help ease body self-consciousness. Say something like, "I know you think your stomach is unattractive, but right now I want you to lie back and allow me to make love to this beautiful belly that you put down so often. You just enjoy the feeling."

Start with parts of their body they're more comfortable with and move slowly in the direction of their neglected area. Ask if they can feel your desire coming through your hands as you caress, stroke, and squeeze them.

Make love to them with words as well: "When I look at you, I see the whole you: this loving, radiant human being. I don't see your belly in isolation. It's just one part of this person I love. When I'm kissing your mouth, it's always wonderful. When I kiss your belly, it's that same wonderful experience for me."

If they're comfortable masturbating, you might even suggest they pleasure themselves while you continue giving that area special attention.

Although it might take time to see progress, it's also possible that if you make love to your partner's belly over a long, sensual evening, that could be all it takes for them to get over their belief that it's not good enough!

Jacob and Brad: Rewriting an Outdated Story

We'd like to share one more real-life example of how a combination of love and eroticism helped to heal someone of a negative self-perception.

When Jacob starting dating Brad, it became clear as things progressed that Brad "was unwilling to remove his shirt in front of me unless the lights were off," Jacob says. "We were having sex but never in full naked view of each other. He didn't take his shirt off at the beach either, saying his fair skin burnt too easily."

When they eventually talked about it, Brad said that very bad acne as a teenager had left him "deformed" by scars.

"He was so ashamed that no one had seen his back since," Jacob says. "He thought it would be too disgusting."

Jacob suspected that Brad's back wasn't "deformed" at all, but Brad "got so upset talking about it that I knew I had to tread lightly," Jacob says. "I would raise the question from time to time, encouraging him to let me touch his back—which he eventually did—and then one day perhaps to even let me see it."

After a few months, Brad finally felt comfortable enough with Jacob to agree.

"It was a big event for him," Jacob recalls, "sitting on the edge of the bed that day, facing away from me toward a window with his head bowed, tearful and afraid of what my reaction was going to be. I promised him that no matter what his back did or didn't look like, there was no way it would affect our relationship. After a while he said he was ready and sick of hiding. In the afternoon light, he ripped off his shirt and threw it on the floor."

Sitting behind him on the bed, Jacob says he saw "nothing remarkable, just a pale-skinned guy sitting with his back to me. I spoke to him about what I could see and stroked and kissed his back. He insisted there were bad scars. I asked him to point to where he thought they were and then I described whatever I could see, which was possibly freckles or just some very tiny remnants of scars. After going over the whole area, we just hung out for a while with his back exposed."

Jacob says that after this reveal, Brad became much more confident.

"He took his shirt off not just with me but in other settings, even telling friends about his years of shame and showing them his back. He got consistent feedback that there was nothing notable about it at all. It was a perfectly fine back. And we were able to have lots more fun together, dancing around naked and being sexually spontaneous."

Jacob's loving, accepting, no-pressure approach had freed Brad of the negative self-perception that had been holding him back his entire adult life.

What Jacob did for Brad is, in essence, a form of narrative therapy. With this counseling technique, a person is helped to identify and rewrite a narrative, or story, that they've been telling themselves, sometimes for decades.

All of us carry around stories we've created about ourselves that can affect how we see ourselves and how we interact with others. For example, suppose that as children we were told we're lazy, or incapable, or have nothing of value to contribute. We will likely take that story with us into adulthood and frequently view ourselves and our life situations through the lens of that story, without ever realizing how much influence it's having on our life and our relationships. A lover can sometimes be the perfect person to help someone identify a destructive narrative, question its validity, and begin to rewrite it.

EROTICIZING SHAME

Joe here. I guess it's my turn.

Like many issues affecting one's ability to be intimate, mine involves a deep-seated sense of shame that's been with me for a long time. I probably had as much shame about a part of my body that

I have absolutely no control over as I have pride about the things I *do* have some control over: my level of fitness, my muscle tone, my physique. In the locker room, it's easy to tell when someone is proud of his package. They're the ones strutting around without a towel and facing out away from the shower! I'm guessing that some of these guys have looked at me and thought, too bad for him.

Then I met Mali.

Before we made love the first time, I shyly confessed to her that I was on the small side, which had occasionally been an issue with lovers in the past—and then quickly reassured her that I had spent considerable time developing other skills. Mali smiled. She explained to me that with almost all of her previous partners, she'd experienced pain following intercourse. Because her vaginal canal is relatively short, the impact against her cervix would cause severe cramping that could last for several hours. She said we just might make a perfect match, and she was right. She loves that I can let go with wild abandon and she almost never experiences pain afterwards.

Knowing this, I can intellectually say that I'm the ideal size for Mali. I also know that statistically I'm actually quite average.[2] In addition, Mali likes to remind me that some well-endowed guys have trouble finding partners who can accommodate them, that smaller is generally better for anal sex, and that there are plenty of heterosexual women like her who actually prefer a small- or average-sized guy.

Finally, I've also come to see the silver lining here: feeling inadequate made me determined to excel at the arts of kissing and oral sex. I've been complimented on my "talented mouth" often enough to know that my dedication paid off!

However, even after almost two decades of truly amazing sex, and with Mali experiencing no end of orgasms through intercourse, I still haven't been able to completely shake this notion that I'm insufficient. My sense of shame has lessened considerably over the years, but every "bigger is better" joke can bring what's left up to the surface again. Although Mali's permanently let go of her belief that the size of her breasts is a problem, I realize that I may never get to the same place. But knowing what I know today, I'm not sure I'd change anything. Not only am I the right size for the woman I love, but my occasional insecurity gives Mali yet another opportunity to try something new to get me a little bit closer to getting over it. In other words, she keeps finding ways to eroticize my size. It may never get any bigger, but you really can't feel too sorry for me for being the subject of all Mali's crazy, loving experiments!

For example, she often embellishes oral sex with "oral sex," telling me she loves how tight, smooth, beautifully shaped, and responsive I am (her words!). She reminds me how much pleasure I've brought her over the years, and that my user-friendly size allows her to do things and create sensations that larger guys would miss out on.

She also has a little trick she calls "conditional head" (I call it blowjob bribery). She goes down on me as long as I focus on knowing that my cock is the perfect size. She'll actually pause periodically and ask, "Can you feel that you are the perfect size?" This sweet sexual torture forces me to fully enjoy her attention. It's a pretty profound experience. Before Mali came along, it was always a challenge to indulge myself in the ecstasy that oral sex can be.

I now know beyond a doubt that our capacity to experience pleasure is greatly increased when we can suspend our "I'm not enough" beliefs, even if only temporarily. In addition, I've learned firsthand that it's difficult for shame and pleasure to coexist, so sucking the shame out of someone, as Mali did, or kissing it out of them, or just loving it out of them really is possible.

It may be of some comfort to realize that almost everyone you know—from your friends and previous partners to politicians, religious leaders, and doctors—suffers from shame too. Men's shame often has an added layer, as they can feel ashamed of even having shame. In part, this is because many people were raised in an environment in which bodies, desires, and sexuality are not okay and beautiful but instead bad, "dirty," or even evil. Showing any weakness, men have been told, means they're not being strong and masculine enough. Almost every story in this chapter—whether about body-image issues, inhibitions, performance anxiety, or the fears surrounding aging—has a component of shame.

Research professor and shame expert Brené Brown says that one of the primary stages of healing shame is being able to talk about it in a safe environment. Bringing your stories out into the open with a partner you trust and receiving their validation, empathy, and compassion will help to dissolve your own feelings of shame. As Brown says, "Shame loses power when it is spoken."[3]

We hope the stories that follow of other couples who used the healing power of eroticism to help dissolve shame will inspire you to come up with your own ideas for working with any shame that you or your partner suffers from. As any sort of sexual or genital shame can be deep and difficult to unravel, enlisting the assistance of someone who specializes in that area, such as a licensed sex counselor, sex therapist, or sexological bodyworker, can be invaluable.

Ask Your Older, Wiser Self

The families or societies in which we were raised are the origin of a lot of body shame. "I was taught growing up that you're not supposed to feel good about yourself, it's narcissistic," explains Latonya. "So I never felt comfortable in my body. When I began to get teased as a teen for having large breasts, I started to crumble. I became very self-conscious and did everything I could to hide them."

If your partner feels shame or embarrassment about some aspect of their body, ask them to imagine themselves twenty or thirty years from now looking back on their body today. What does their older, wiser self have to say about the negative thoughts they're having? When she viewed her feminine curves through the eyes of sixty-year-old Latonya, her older and much wiser self emphatically declared, "You are a lovely woman with a voluptuous, feminine figure. Stop obsessing, and start living it up with those!"

Own Your Lusty Self

The safety and support of an intimate relationship can empower someone to take a risk and embody an aspect of themselves they've been ashamed of. Gail was raised in a household where sex was a bad word. "I learned growing up that if you like sex, you're a slut. If you enjoy flirting, you're a prick-tease." She was always told to "dress like a lady," meaning she had to keep her shoulders and thighs covered, while her friends wore strapless tops and miniskirts. For years she felt guilty and sinful about her sexuality. But with her husband Calvin's reassurance and support, she has slowly allowed her lascivious side to come out and play.

Calvin started by encouraging her to wear provocative outfits at home. Eventually Gail felt freer about her fashion choices outside the house. "My shoulders are one of my best features. No more hiding them!" she laughs. Halloween, when she can fully embrace her "lusty woman persona," has become their favorite holiday. "I still feel like I'm being a 'bad girl,'" Gail says, "but now instead of being ashamed about it, I have fun with it!"

Turn It into a Sexy Story

If one of you feels shame around a past experience, there's sometimes a way to create something positive out of those memories.

"Kate slept with a lot of guys in college, and even though she had fun at the time, she's not especially proud of that period in her life," says Jack. "But I actually love hearing about her experiences. I can imagine her starring in all these sexy roles!"

At first Kate was very resistant to telling her husband the specifics about her college escapades, "because of the shame I felt about being labeled a 'campus slut'," she says. But over the years, with Jack's patient, loving encouragement, she's discovered that sharing these stories with the man who's crazy about her, and even elaborating on the details, is actually healing because "something good is coming out of those embarrassing memories."

Use Erotica for Healing

Almost anything we can feel sexual shame around—like the perception of having a smaller- or larger-than-average body part, feeling over- or underweight, or having scars—is something that other people (very often *many* other people) view as a turn-on. And anything that many people view as a turn-on is going to be featured in visual and written erotica. There are sites that focus entirely on anything from having prominent or abundant veins, wrinkles, freckles, or body hair to being unusually tall or short. If you, or you and your partner together, are comfortable searching for erotica focused on your particular "issue," you might come across sites whose mere existence tells you that it *is* possible to see this aspect of yourself as sexually desirable.

As Carla entered her forties, for example, she started feeling shame for being older, which began to inhibit her sexually. Eventually she discovered erotica featuring MILFs ("mothers I'd like to fuck") and "cougars" (referring to experienced women who date younger men), in which older women are the objects of desire. Their age gives them an aura of sexual expertise and confidence. "Reading stories featuring women who are attractive and sexy precisely *because* they're older helps me to see myself that way as well," Carla says.

As another example of a couple who used erotica in a healing context, Oscar has always been self-conscious about the facial expressions he makes when having an orgasm. Then his lover came across a site focused exclusively on showcasing the real, unrestrained pleasure on people's faces during sex, and the couple spent some time looking through the photos and videos. "Even if I still think my face looks weird sometimes," Oscar says, "it's reassuring to know there are people who enjoy seeing what it *really* looks like when people come. It helps me stop worrying about what my face is doing."

Play with the Fantasy

As a self-protective mechanism, our minds occasionally eroticize incidences from our past that we experienced as shameful or traumatic.[4] For example, a child who was made to feel ashamed of their naked body might, as an adult, find themselves turned on by thoughts of being naked in public.

If fantasies like these make us feel conflicted or confused, it helps to understand that our imagination sometimes gets involved as a way of gaining a sense of control over those events. Having the fantasy doesn't mean it's something we would ever want to happen in real life. Instead, by allowing us to play with those situations and themes while being in complete control of everything that's occurring—it's not happening against your will when it's *your* fantasy—fantasies like these can be quite therapeutic. In addition, sharing such a fantasy with a loving partner can be both healing and empowering.

Kathryn had always been disturbed by her fantasies of being spanked, which she'd had since she was quite young. One weekend, she finally felt comfortable enough to confess these fantasies to Robin, her partner of many years.

After talking about it for a few weeks, they decided to play out a simple spanking scenario. Kathryn not only found herself tremendously turned on, but "after all those years it lost some of its hold over me," she says. "Robin made it fun and silly, and I suddenly didn't feel nearly as ashamed." She feels very fortunate that "now it's something Robin and I can explore safely." Playing with this scenario together allowed Kathryn to make a lasting shift in how she feels about having these fantasies.

Play Out a New Ending

Role-play is often used in therapeutic settings to help someone work through an incident from their past. This could be a time they were talked into doing something they didn't want to do, touched in a way they didn't like, or criticized for their body or their sexual performance. This is another approach that lovers can use to help each other transform their relationship with a past experience.

For example, you might role-play with your partner an event they still feel troubled or embarrassed about, such as a time they were kissed without their consent. Re-creating the scenario gives them a chance to practice responding differently, to be strong in that situation instead of acquiescing, to say no clearly and emphatically. Don't let a fear of acting hold you back. The focus is not on how well you act, but on the conversations and healing insights that arise.

It also may be possible to use role-playing in a loving, consensual context, and involve the assistance of a trained counselor or psychologist, to help a lover reframe a seriously distressing experience, such as sexual assault.

Celebrate Your Uniqueness

Humans have a natural affinity for symmetry, which is one reason why some women don't like the look of their vulvas. In pornography, we see airbrushed and surgically sanitized female genitalia that become further removed from reality with every technological advancement.

Dani, who's in her late twenties, was actually saving up for labiaplasty (vulva surgery) until she started dating Marcus, a professional body piercer. When she confessed her embarrassment that her left labia was longer and fuller than her right, making her feel lopsided, he said, "I've seen everything, and your vulva's asymmetry doesn't make it ugly. It makes it unique!" Natural vulvas, he told her, are all different (in fact, in real life, asymmetrical labia are more common than not). Marcus told Dani that he truly appreciated the variation. So instead of surgery, she went with jewelry. Marcus did a piercing on her shorter lip to create an artistically balanced look. With all the lovely jewelry made for adorning vulvas, Dani will never run out of beautiful ways to celebrate her uniqueness.

A similar example of celebrating one's uniqueness is breast cancer survivors who have elaborate tattoos created over their mastectomy scars. This permanent body art helps some people embrace their new bodies by transforming what they previously viewed as disfigurement into beauty.

If the pain and healing time of an actual piercing or tattoo doesn't appeal to you, there are plenty of clip-on jewelry and temporary tattoo options designed especially for vulvas, nipples, navels, and penises—anything you have an issue with that could benefit from a little reminder to accept and appreciate the beautiful, asymmetrical you.

In Celebration of Vulva Variation

I (Joe) would like to take this opportunity to emphasize again that variation is something to be celebrated, not "corrected." Labiaplasty is one of the fastest-growing cosmetic surgeries in the world, yet it often involves taking something uniquely beautiful and making it generic by removing its individuality.

There are physical or functional reasons for labiaplasty, such as discomfort during sex or exercise and trauma to the tissues caused during childbirth. However, the majority of surgeries today are performed for aesthetic reasons. Surgery typically involves trimming the inner lips (labia minora) to rest inside the outer lips (labia majora) to make things look smoother and more symmetrical.

Countless women are having this elective surgery because they believe their vulvas are "ugly" or "weird." This belief is often the result of exposure to the sanitized images perpetuated by porn, and perhaps even to the profusion of before-and-after photos on plastic surgery websites. Additionally, women may have heard negative comments about their own vulvas from other people—people who have been similarly brainwashed.

It's helpful here to point out, as obstetrician-gynecologist Jen Gunter explains in *The Vagina Bible*, that "50 percent of women have labia minora that protrude beyond the labia majora, and yet 75 percent of women who are built this way think it is abnormal."

For some women who feel they will never be able to see their very normal vulvas as beautiful, the psychological benefit of surgery might be just as important as the physical benefit for someone who is in pain. However, if you or someone you know is considering labiaplasty for aesthetic reasons, I'd like you to consider another perspective.

Vulvas are as unique as faces. Even within a single woman, variation is normal. A woman's vulva can look different depending on whether she's feeling warm or chilly; whether she's been sitting, walking, or lying down; or whether she's had panties pressed up against her for a while or is fresh out of the shower. When things *aren't* symmetrical, or when the inner labia *do* protrude, there are more possibilities for playful (and pleasurable!) exploration. There's less to discover if everything's been "tidied up"! And if the inner labia have an edge that's darker than the rest of the labia (another reason women sometimes opt for surgery), that color variation can easily be seen as an enchanting artistic embellishment.

So don't let porn or plastic-surgery infomercials shame you into believing that all vulvas should look a certain way. This doesn't just apply to people with vulvas. It's also for those who are lucky enough to make love to them! Your partner will be more relaxed and receptive when she knows you accept and appreciate her just as she is. Take time to savor the intricacies and uniqueness of her body. You'll both have a more enjoyable experience.

So many utopian novels and movies portray a future in which everyone has been made essentially the same, yet it's the renegades, those who have somehow escaped the treatments and therapies to make them conform, that are the desirable ones. When we get tired of striving for someone else's idea of perfection, we'll realize that we can see perfection wherever we choose to.

EROTICIZING INHIBITIONS

Over a weeklong camping trip when he was a senior in high school, Daniel snuck into his girlfriend's tent while her tent mate was out with *her* boyfriend. Tess and Daniel had both been looking forward to this, as it was the first time they were going to try oral sex. But for Daniel, the smell and taste were so strong that he just couldn't bring himself to try it again.

This aversion sexually inhibited him until law school, where he met Allison. When he admitted he wasn't crazy about cunnilingus, Allison asked for the details.

"She was so matter-of-fact about it," he recalls. "She told me, 'Your first pussy was probably just a little overripe from camping too long without a shower.'" Allison told Daniel that the scent of a vagina is supposed to be an aphrodisiac and that there was nothing at all wrong with his girlfriend's vagina.

"'Let me tell you what it's like to eat fresh pussy,' she told me. She described it so sensuously that I was practically drooling!" Allison's erotic description was just the enticement Daniel needed to give oral another try.

Daniel, now a cunnilingus connoisseur, smiles and says that Allison was right. "Vaginas smell and taste like women and sex," he says. "That combination is intoxicating!"

Because of the abundance of negative messages out there about vaginas, and the unnecessary and potentially harmful products like deodorants and douches marketed to women, I (Joe) want to add that a well-seasoned vagina can be a real turn-on. And if you've just returned home from a week of backpacking, so can sensuously washing each other down before indulging in the evening's oral treats! In addition, as sex therapist Ian Kerner points out in *She Comes First: The Thinking Man's Guide to Pleasuring a Woman*, "a woman's genitals are a self-cleaning system—more sanitary than many other parts of the body, including the mouth."

Inhibitions can be brought on not only by negative experiences, but by negative messages or misinformation about sex we received while growing up.

Leslie and her boyfriend of seven years have a great sex life. Wanting to keep it that way, one day Leslie suggested checking out some sex toys. Dave was less than enthusiastic. Knowing him as well as she did, Leslie recognized his hesitation as just part of his general reluctance to trying something new. So rather than being deterred, she put her mind to thinking of ways they could have a low-key encounter with a sex toy or two. As Dave was a precision machinist and an avid reader of *Popular Mechanics*, Leslie had a suspicion he might find the design and construction of the first vibrators interesting. She found an informative website on the history of sex toys, and they had a fun time looking through the old photos, product descriptions, and hilarious advertisements together.

A couple of weeks later, in anticipation of her birthday, Leslie mischievously mentioned that she'd always wondered about benwa balls, which were popular in the eighties when she was growing up. "We could pick out a pair at that fancy adult store downtown," she suggested with a smile, "and you could help me put them in place!" Dave had never heard of benwa balls, but he found this an intriguing proposition.

Instead of just a quick in-and-out to procure the benwa balls, the gleam of the titanium butt plugs on display caught Dave's eye as they entered the store, and the couple spent half an hour speaking with the sales assistant about the pros and cons of the various models and materials. Now the expert, Dave went on about the advantages of steel versus glass versus silicone all the way home. Their adventures into the world of sex toys had begun!

Here are several common situations where a little eroticism between lovers can not only help free someone from a sexual inhibition but even have profound healing effects. As you read these accounts, notice these recurring themes:

- Approach the inhibition from creative new angles.
- Move at the pace of the partner with the inhibition (no rushing!).
- Be generous with the empathy and reassurance.

You might also consider talking to a counselor about other ways to help lessen an inhibition, whether yours or your partner's.

Help Them Erotically Own It

An inhibition that keeps us from feeling comfortable in our body can sometimes be helped by a slow, gentle shift of perspective.

For instance, George really wanted to see his girlfriend Sharise braless out in public, but she had never liked the idea. When they talked about it, he learned that she felt "too sexual" or "slutty" when people could see the outline of her breasts or her nipples through her shirt. She was, however, willing to try going without a bra around their apartment, when it was just the two of them. She felt surprisingly comfortable with that, so she agreed to go a step further and wear a shirt in which she didn't look braless out on a date. No one else knew, but *they* did, and there was something erotic about sharing this secret.

At home, George encouraged Sharise to try on a couple of different tops and notice how the fabric felt against her bare breasts. She had to admit that it felt good. He then asked her to "stand tall and walk like you own them," which made her laugh at first but really did give her a sense of confidence. Sharise began to associate being braless with fun sexy times with her husband instead of with her old idea that people would think she was a slut.

When she was finally ready to go out to a dark club in a thin top that didn't hide what she was up to, George told Sharise to remember that he was loving it.

"If I find myself thinking, what will people think?" she says now, "I remind myself that our opinions are the only two that matter!"

Entice Them with Brief Encounters

Francesca, a reformed Catholic, says her hottest fantasy is to "make love in forbidden places." She finally worked up the courage to tell her boyfriend about it, but the prospect made him very uneasy.

The scariest part, she learned from Andrew, is that they might get in trouble. So Francesca playfully suggested a few things they could do that had the flavor of being in a public place but no danger of getting caught: stealing a kiss in a secluded corner of a dark restaurant, making out in the car down a dead-end road, having sex in a hotel at night with the curtains open but the room lights turned off. Andrew was willing to give it a try, because the nervousness he felt around these suggestions felt manageable enough to interpret as exciting. By finding enticing ways for Andrew to feel comfortable exploring "forbidden places" with her, *her* fantasy eventually became *their* fantasy—as well as their reality.

Eroticize Fears in Fantasy

Kiara started dating a man who, like her, was interested in exploring bondage. The first time was a little scary but very exciting. The second time, though, he went too far, pushing her past what she'd said she was ready for and leaving her feeling abused and afraid. It took her months before she even felt like dating again.

Then Kiara met Steve. Eventually she felt close enough to tell him about those experiences, and he was appalled at how she'd been treated. Steve said he'd never been into bondage, but he was into her—and was up for exploring her desires at whatever pace was comfortable for her. So far, they've just had sexy conversations about all the things he's "going to do to her."

"Even that can feel very intense," Kiara says. "I'm at my edge, though it's a psychological edge rather than a physical edge."

Kiara and Steve may or may not take their explorations any further, but either way, their erotic conversations—and the real trust they are developing by Steve respecting her feelings and honoring her boundaries—are helping Kiara heal from the trauma she'd suffered.

Make a New Erotic Association

If we're inhibited because we've linked a smell, pain, or a feeling of embarrassment to a particular sex act or position, eroticism can be a way to unlink these things. This is what Allison did when she helped Daniel separate the act of going down on a woman from his memory of a particular smell and associate it instead with a sensual description of what cunnilingus *could* be like.

Christie and her husband John took a similar approach in helping Christie reclaim her breasts as objects of desire after two children and four continuous years of breastfeeding. When they first embarked on this journey, John said to Christie, "You may not be able to see them as sexual right now, but I can!" He told her he was happy to just enjoy looking at them whenever the couple made love, and to wait until she decided she was ready—however long that might take—before he touched them again.

Eventually Christie felt comfortable enough to pick out a couple of beautiful bras to wear when they made love, and the couple sometimes positioned themselves so they could both view her chest in a mirror. John would frequently tell her how sexy it was just to watch her, which helped Christie begin to reclaim an erotic connection with her breasts. John says that Christie's breasts being off limits for all that time "made me crave them even more. It was a year-long perpetual turn-on!" Slowly re-involving her breasts in a sexual context with her husband helped Christie eventually allow them to once again be objects of pleasure and desire.

Offer a Loving Invitation

Here's one of our own stories of how connecting—and fun!—it can be to help the one you love let go of an inhibition. When I (Joe) first met Mali, I was quite nervous about being naked in the presence of other people. I probably looked at her in mock horror when she suggested we take a trip to a clothing-optional hot springs. The idea actually appealed to me. I put on shorts the first day of spring, and I like being naked at home, especially hanging out with Mali on our deck. And the thought of getting to the point of feeling comfortable around others was a draw. Not only that, it was something exciting for us to try together.

A previous partner had once tried to get me to visit the same hot springs: "What's the big deal?" she snapped at me when I expressed reservations. "You just take your towel off!" Her approach—no empathy, no reassurance, no support—definitely didn't inspire, and we never made that happen. From her I learned the sure-fire way *not* to get your partner to try something new: by shaming them into it! And from Mali I've learned the method that has the *best* chance of encouraging someone to try something new: an enticing, no-pressure invitation.

We went for a weekend. At first we found a natural pool away from the other guests, where we could just get comfortable ourselves, together, before venturing out onto the decks where most of the people hung out. Mali encouraged me to focus on the sensual feeling of the sun and water on my skin, and on the beauty of the nature around us, rather than on worrying about being judged or comparing myself to others. I had to admit that I liked the feeling of being outdoors with nothing on, and I loved seeing Mali so at ease naked.

I wasn't quite so comfortable the first time I walked around in the more public space without a towel around my waist. I was trying to keep a low profile, but the first couple who saw us burst out with, "Look at that guy's *tan*!" We had to laugh. From my decades as a competitive swimmer, there was a stark color contrast between the rest of my body and the area Mali affectionately calls my "birthday Speedo."

A dozen pairs of eyes were momentarily drawn to the narrow band of white skin around my hips. I began to relax when I realized no one was whispering or snickering, no one was pointing and laughing. It just took time and, well, exposure for me to let go of my self-created inhibitions and enjoy the freedom—and sexiness!—of being naked outdoors with the love of my life.

EROTICIZING PERFORMANCE ANXIETY

In addition to helping with negative self-perceptions, inhibitions, and feelings of shame or embarrassment, a little eroticism is a natural way to help ease performance anxiety. People often think that only men have this concern. But anyone who is held back by fears of whether their partner will think they're good in bed, how their body might respond sexually, or if they'll be able to reach orgasm has performance anxiety.

After dating for several weeks and before having sex for the first time, Ann and Thomas both revealed that they felt some trepidation, as neither had been in a relationship for a number of years. Thomas, a widower busy with two teenagers, was concerned about his ability to get and maintain an erection. Ann, having entered menopause since the last time she'd had sex with a partner, was worried she might have an issue with lubrication. In essence, they were both feeling anxious about their future performance.

They decided they would both invest in a little bedside reassurance. Ann did some research and chose a personal lubricant. Thomas requested a prescription for Viagra from his doctor. Not only did their preparations relieve the performance pressure they were feeling, but "revealing these things to each other was so intimate," says Ann. They tell the story with a laugh, because six months' worth of lovemaking later, neither of them had even opened their purchases.

Mind over Love Muscle

Issues with getting or maintaining an erection are the most obvious manifestations of performance anxiety. Many couples regard any type of erectile inconsistency or dysfunction as a problem, even though it's common enough that it's more like "normal" function than "dys" function![5] Although there are sometimes physiological reasons for erectile issues, including high blood pressure, diabetes, smoking, and taking certain prescription medications, the cause is quite often psychological.

Suppose that Justin, for example, doesn't want his new girlfriend going down on him because of previous problems with losing his erection. In situations like this, performance anxiety often becomes a self-fulfilling prophecy. During oral sex, Justin may very well be unable to maintain an erection precisely because he's worried about maintaining an erection.

If, however, Justin is able to talk about what's going on for him, his new girlfriend could focus on creating an environment free of pressure. She could explain that she understands there isn't always a link between arousal and erection and that she's not going to interpret any absence of erection as meaning that Justin doesn't find her sexy or attractive. She could reassure him that she will enjoy going down on him whether or not he gets erect, because her intention is simply to explore all the different pleasurable sensations she can create in whatever state of arousal his penis happens to be in. She could also tell him that even if he does get hard, it's more than okay if he loses his erection, because of the fun she'll have trying to tease it back again!

Conditional Head

The little trick we mentioned earlier is useful for all kinds of performance anxiety, including issues with erections and ejaculation control. The concept is simple. If your lover is anxious about getting or keeping an erection, tell them you will focus your oral attentions on them as long as they don't get hard. The moment you feel them start to respond, you'll slow down or move on to something else until they're soft again. The purpose of this "healing head" is for them to fully enjoy your love and attention, not to become erect.

I (Mali) discovered this trick when I was dating a man who regularly ejaculated before he wanted to. Intercourse or fellatio typically lasted ten or twenty seconds at most. One Saturday morning, I decided I would do whatever I could to help him last longer. I started by going down on him, but if I felt he was getting too stimulated, I'd pull away. I also required him to keep up a continual commentary on everything I was doing ("You're running your hand along my right thigh, now you're squeezing my hip"), which helped divert some of his attention away from what was happening in his genitals. Later, I told him we could only have intercourse for half a minute at a time. If it went on any longer than that, he would have to pull out and wait a while. By that evening, after several hours of this "conditional coitus," he was able to last far longer during intercourse than he ever had before.[6]

A similar approach might be helpful for someone who can't relax during cunnilingus because they're worried that they won't climax. You simply tell them you will pleasure them only as long as they *don't* come! This technique can help move someone's attention away from worry and fear and into what they're feeling in their body.

Try Some Erotic Experimentation

When Takira met Matt, she made a decision. Even though she had often faked orgasms in the past, usually so that her partner would feel that he was a good lover, she didn't want to start up that habit again. So instead she told Matt the truth: that she was able to have an orgasm on her own but had never had one with a partner.

The issue wasn't that Takira thought she should be able to orgasm from intercourse alone. She knew that only around 25 percent of women do that with any regularity.[7] She had never had an orgasm through any kind of stimulation from a lover, whether with his hands, his mouth, or his penis.

Takira's experience is not uncommon. In situations where a woman can orgasm on her own, there's obviously no physical reason why she shouldn't be able to orgasm with a partner. Frequently, women who have this difficulty feel self-conscious about their body, their genitals, or the type of stimulation they need and are uncomfortable communicating about the topic. They may be concerned that their orgasm will require "too much" of their partner's time and attention or that their partner might get bored. Or they might be preoccupied with how they look or what their partner is thinking about.

Takira hit the jackpot when she found Matt. "He said to me, 'Let's explore all kinds of things as we search for your orgasm. We might find it together, or we might not, but we'll sure have a fun time trying!'" Matt's idea of turning her elusive orgasm into an incentive for experimenting, Takira says, took the pressure off instantly.

If you find yourself in a similar situation—able to orgasm on your own but not with a partner—take a deep dive together into exploring motions, pressure, and sensations, which could be a tremendous turn-on for you both. You can experiment with all kinds of stimulation, whether that's with their hands, their mouth, or toys. Try different positions and different kinds of touch—rubbing, pressing, tapping, light, slow, firm, fiery. Vary what you yourself do too, such as focusing your attention on the stimulation you're receiving or on a fantasy you enjoy. Try both relaxing your muscles and tensing them. Although women who have difficulty climaxing are often advised to relax their bodies, some need to do just the opposite.

If you're comfortable masturbating while your partner watches, let them see exactly what works for you as you self-pleasure. If you're too self-conscious for that, you could pleasure yourself with your partner nearby but the lights lowered or with them holding you from behind. If you fantasize when you masturbate, you might share your fantasy with your partner so they can be involved with that part of your experience. Or take your lover's hands and use them as you would your own hands.

If you're the one helping your partner, reassure them that they don't need to worry about whether you're having a good time. Orgasm exploration, with the goal of discovery, intimacy, and pleasure, is anything but boring. They may need reassurance more than once that if they don't come, now or ever, you won't be disappointed. An accepting, adventurous attitude on your part just might help set their elusive orgasm free!

Beginner's Mind

Performance anxiety can have its origins in a previous experience, such as someone who was once told they were a bad kisser or not good at sex. The Zen Buddhist practice of having an open or "beginner's" mind, free of preconceptions and judgments, can work wonders here.

If one of you believes you're "bad" at a particular sexual activity, approach it as though neither of you has ever done the activity before. You are both beginners, experimenting and learning together.

Set Your Voice Free

The first two years I (Mali) was sexually active, I never once had an orgasm with a partner, only on my own. One night, while having intercourse with my boyfriend of several months, I decided to fake it and just pretend I was having one—and something amazing happened. I started to come for real!

I understand now why this worked. Up until that day, I'd always held myself back from making noise during sex, but sound is one of the body's natural ways of expressing itself. Sound is stimulating, and vocalizing your pleasure helps your partner sense and respond to your level of excitement. Letting myself make noise freed up something I had been holding back. It excited me to sound like that, and I could tell my boyfriend was excited by it too.

I'm not recommending that you start faking orgasms—there are plenty of reasons why *that's* a bad idea—but you might want to start playing around with being a little more vocal in bed.

If your lover has difficulty reaching orgasm, it's possible that they're censoring their sounds—or movements or facial expressions—because they think you'll find them strange or repulsive. Reassuring them that any authentic sounds they make are going to sound erotic to you might just give them the freedom to *really* let go!

ADVENTURES IN AGING

It's not uncommon for older people to say that they find sex more meaningful, intimate, and fulfilling than when they were younger. Along with not having to worry about birth control, they talk about feeling more relaxed with who they are, less self-conscious, and more comfortable with their bodies. We've heard from numerous couples in their forties, fifties, sixties, and even seventies who are having the best sex of their lives.

"I don't think I could have had this kind of relationship in my twenties or thirties," says Sandy. "I was too hung up on what other people thought of me—and what I thought of myself. At our age, we don't take each other or the relationship for granted." And Carmen says, "When you fall in love later in life, there's a feeling that you've turned back the clock, while also being appreciative of the limited time you have together."

In *Magnificent Sex: Lessons from Extraordinary Lovers*, researchers Peggy J. Kleinplatz and A. Dana Ménard conducted extensive interviews in a quest to discover what makes sex magnificent. A substantial proportion of their interviewees were individuals over the age of 60 who had been in a relationship for 25 years or longer. The authors identified eight universal components of extraordinary sexual experiences as described by the participants:

1. The feeling of being completely present and absorbed in the moment
2. The feeling of being fully connected and in sync with one's partner
3. Deep feelings of sexual and erotic intimacy, trust, and mutual respect
4. Extraordinary verbal and nonverbal communication, a willingness to fully share bodies and souls, and feelings of deep empathy
5. Being completely authentic, honest, and self-revealing
6. Being vulnerable and emotionally naked, completely letting go
7. Exploring and discovering self and other, expanding personal boundaries, and having a sense of play, fun, and humor
8. Transcendence (experiencing heightened mental, emotional, physical, spiritual, and relational states) and transformation (having life-affirming, growth-enhancing, and life-altering experiences)

Note that none of these components has anything to do with bodies, techniques, positions, or sexual performance—meaning magnificent sex is accessible to us at any age!

Discover the Art in Aging

In *Better Than I Ever Expected: Straight Talk About Sex After Sixty*, senior sex expert Joan Price writes, "Loving and appreciating our bodies goes hand in hand with having joyful sex." See each other as the continually evolving works of art that you are by looking at your lover's face—the familiar features, the lines, the things that have changed since you first met—in the same way you would look at a sculpture or painting. Do the same for yourself, looking in the mirror and reflecting on the truth that all your life experiences—the everyday ones, the challenging ones, and the amazing ones—had a hand in shaping this unique work of art before you.

Natasha and Christian met in their late fifties. "Curiosity can be a good starting point for learning about each other's past," Natasha says. "We once spent an evening telling the stories behind the marks on our bodies: my restructured nipple after breast surgery, the burn mark on his arm, the small half-moon scar on a finger. Appreciating your lover's history as etched on their skin gives you insight into what has shaped them into who they are today."

Rhonda and Dean, who raised three children together, say they practice seeing each other as spiritual beings in human bodies who are going through the normal aging process. "When I look at Dean and feel that spiritual part of him," says Rhonda, "it's as though he hasn't aged at all, no matter how much his body might have changed."

Talk to Yourselves with Love

Everywhere we turn, we're bombarded by negative stereotypes and perceptions about intimacy and aging: "Sex is for the young and beautiful." "Old is ugly. Youth is sexy." "No one's going to want you when you're old." By the time we start to feel our age, these messages are often deeply ingrained.

If you are burdened with beliefs like these, some conscious reprogramming is in order. Start by reminding yourself, "I'm experienced—

and experience is sexy!" Or, "These wrinkles are evidence that I've been through a lot—which means I have a lot to offer." Or simply, "Being older is an attractive quality." Don't believe that last one? Consider the fact that hundreds of thousands of people search daily for pornography with tags like "older," "mature," "cougar," or "MILF" or prefer their porn to feature actors in their forties, fifties, and sixties rather than teenagers or twenty-somethings.[8] If you have a willing partner, you can reinforce positive messages like these by reminding each other, "We can experience pleasure and connection at any age!"

Channel Fear into Action

As people age, it's common to worry about the changes to come: "How will I feel? Will my partner or other people still find me attractive? Will I be able to perform, get an erection, lubricate, get turned on? Will I even have the desire?"

Take the energy you might otherwise expend on worries like these and channel it into doing whatever you can to keep yourself feeling as healthy as possible. Exercising, eating well, helping a friend, and volunteering will all help you to continue feeling vibrant and alive.

Keep on Dancing

To stay strong and flexible, your body needs to be moved, stretched, and challenged. If we can't convince you to try some kind of dance, which can do wonders to keep you feeling fluid and flexible (and, dare we say it, sexy!), do give your body the gift of some sort of movement every day, even if it's just a quick walk around the neighborhood. Many people have limitations when it comes to moving and exercising, but there's always *something* you can do. And if you want to boost your libido, plenty of studies show that physical activity and having sex are two of the best ways. "Physicality," says Joan Price in *Better Than I Ever Expected*, "is a tremendous turn-on."

We know as well as anyone how much intention and effort it takes to do what we can to stay flexible, drink enough water, moderate the drugs and alcohol, and get sufficient rest. But taking on this challenge together, and being each other's support system, is motivating. We're committed to doing everything we can to stay healthy, active, and engaged with life: exercising together, treating our bodies well, continuing to grow emotionally, pursuing creative endeavors, and oh yes—having spirited sex! It's all worth it. It keeps us very attracted to each other, and we have tremendous appreciation for each other's efforts as well.

Activate Those Feel-Good Hormones

Touching, hugging, and kissing can all trigger the release of the hormones dopamine, oxytocin, and serotonin. Known fondly as the pleasure hormone, the love hormone, and the happy hormone respectively, this powerful trio strengthens feelings of affection, empathy, bonding, trust, and attachment. These hormones also affect neuroplasticity, which is the brain's ability to form new connections (required when learning a new skill or language), recover from injury (such as a stroke), and retain knowledge.

The problem is, levels of all three of these hormones fall as we age. Their decrease is associated with declines in everything from cognitive and motor functioning to the regeneration and repair of nerve and muscle cells.

One way to help keep the levels of these feel-good hormones higher is to hug, touch, and kiss more often. If you pay attention, you might notice the effects of these behaviors immediately. Just from kissing, says fifty-seven-year-old Melissa, "I can feel the levels rise. Then they go down again, and after a while I need another hit!" In addition, offering each other little massages here and there will not only keep these helpful hormones circulating, but also help alleviate stiffness and tension.

Be Open to Options

The sex lives of countless couples are negatively affected by common physical changes like erection inconsistencies and vaginal dryness. Don't be afraid to talk to your health care provider about any changes you notice. And if they seem uncomfortable talking to *you* about sexual issues, find another provider! Do try the remedies recommended to you if you need them. That's what they're there for. There's no shame in using a medication (such as Cialis, Viagra, or Levitra) or other treatments for ED (erectile dysfunction). If you're experiencing vaginal dryness, there are supplements and personal lubricants (which are different from standard sex lube) that could help, as well as estrogen creams and suppositories (if you and your doctor decide they are a good choice for you). Invest in a vibrator if you're finding you need more stimulation than you used to.

Even if none of the available options work for you, it's still possible to have sexually intimate and loving experiences. Mark is in his late sixties and can no longer get erections following medical treatment for prostate cancer. He isn't a candidate for erectile aids such as vacuum pumps, injections, or implants, nor will a cock ring (which can help a penis stay hard) or a sleeve (a hollow, typically silicone penis that goes over one's own) work for him. And yet, he and his wife Ellen still enjoy their sexual connection. "It's true, we can no longer have intercourse the traditional way," Ellen says, "but there are lots of things we *can* do, enough to keep us busy for a long time!" As Mark and Ellen can attest, satisfying sex does not require an erect penis.

Reconnect with Your Passion from the Past

If your libido's been lacking, try this little trick. Think back to when you were younger and had a serious crush, when just brushing arms was electrifying. Call up the scenarios you used to run through your mind, and see if you can generate some of those feelings of longing and desire again. For me (Mali), imagining myself back in eighth grade secretly watching my science teacher play tetherball in his white Levis does it every time!

Cultivate Desire

If you want your partner to continue to *be* sexy, keep seeing them *as* sexy. Actively look for what you find attractive about them, every day. The "Sweet & Sexy Sixty" photobook I (Mali) made for Joe's sixtieth birthday is a great illustration of this. I love taking pictures of him when I see something I like, capturing those moments for myself. I put many of them together in a book so Joe (and all our friends and family!) could see this beautiful man through my eyes. Joe says from personal experience that when someone *sees* you as attractive, you *feel* more attractive.

Over time, it's natural to stop noticing aspects of the person we're with, even those we really enjoy. So remind yourself of what you are attracted to when you look at your partner: "She has such beautiful hair! I love running my fingers through it." "I just love his hands, so masculine and sensitive—perfect for squeezing me just right!"

In *The Erotic Mind*, sex therapist Jack Morin talks about the idea that remaining attracted to a long-term partner is a choice. "The ability to sustain attraction is, to a significant degree, a conscious decision, an act of will," he says. "It is your responsibility to be actively receptive, to open your eyes enthusiastically to the beauty of your lover."[9]

Another way to cultivate desire is to recall stories of sexy times you've shared in the past, whether that's remembering them yourself or sharing those memories with your lover: "I was just thinking about that time we rented that little cabin on the lake. Especially the fun we had with that outdoor shower!" And dream up some new fantasies for yourself in which they play a starring role.

Also try telling yourself a story about the sex you're going to have later: "The next time we have this house to ourselves, we're going to make out in the living room like a couple of teenagers!" Or, "I can't wait until the next time this man makes love to me. I'm going to be sure to appreciate every moment of that!" Or, "I can't wait until the next time I get to make love to this man!" Or, "I'm looking forward to that special trick she does with her tongue." Or, "I'm looking forward to trying that idea for oral sex that I read about in chapter 3!" Telling yourself something like this will not only cultivate desire for your partner—your partner is likely to feel the seductive energy in the air.

Make Love to the Passage of Time

Here's an out-of-the-ordinary date night idea just for older couples. To prepare, choose several photos from when you each were younger and settle in for the evening.

One by one, really look at each image of your partner. Talk about where the picture was taken, what was happening, and how your partner felt about themselves and the situation. Get a sense of who they were at each of these various moments in their life. As you kiss your partner and make love to them that evening, feel into the person in the photos, connecting with who they were then.

This isn't about not appreciating who your lover is today, as their younger self is *part* of who they are today. It's about sharing aspects of yourselves from the past to create a uniquely fun and connecting experience in the present, which can be healing as well as intimate.

Joe, for example, looks at pictures of himself from his early twenties and sees a very self-conscious guy, a guy who was too shy to even talk to a girl. He just didn't feel confident in himself. On the other hand I (Mali) see a younger version of the man I adore: "You're exactly the type of guy I would have gone crazy over back then!" I tell him. Seeing himself through the eyes of someone who's in love with him has given him quite a different perspective on himself back then.

In the Eye of the Beholder

Not surprisingly, since ageism in our culture disproportionately affects women, I (Mali) have a tougher time than Joe does when it comes to accepting my own aging face. When I can't see beyond the newest spot or wrinkle, this sweet guy helps me find ways to accept the person looking back at me in the mirror.

"You can keep thinking about your wrinkles, or you can focus on the fact that you have the energy and enthusiasm of someone much younger, and you take great care of yourself," Joe will remind me. He'll ask me how old I feel, and I always have to agree that if I didn't know how old I was, I'd guess a lot younger. He'll say things like, "Your passion for life inspires people of all ages" or "Your body has brought me more pleasure over the years than I can possibly even remember" or "These lines on your face are a celebration of your life" or "There's no one else I'd rather get old with." Joe says it doesn't matter what I'm doing, whether I'm sweaty, frowning, or exhausted, he can always see and feel my essence, which he says is a warm, inviting radiance. "The beauty that radiates from within you is timeless, the kind of beauty that doesn't fade," he says. "It's my ongoing mission in life to get you to see what I see: a beautiful, ageless woman." What a sweetie.

When we get really old, he says, we'll get body paints and have a blast painting our wrinkles crazy colors!

From my (Joe's) perspective, age just isn't important. I can see the beauty in women in their twenties and thirties and forties. I can also see the beauty in women in their fifties, sixties, and seventies. And that beauty typically runs deeper, as older women often have a greater depth of experience and are more comfortable with themselves. When I look at Mali, I don't see an aging woman, I see an amazing woman! If your partner, like almost everyone else on the planet, worries from time to time about getting older, read again those things I say to Mali and feel free to use or adapt them to offer your partner some positive reassurance.

We're all aging, all the time. How you choose to respond to aging won't change the inevitability of it, but it will immensely affect your experience of it. We've decided that we might as well approach aging as an adventure, because that attitude is so much better than the alternative!

The older we get, the more we realize how precious every moment we have together is. We are honored and excited to be with each other as we age, to be a witness to the changes, insights, and personal transformations to come. And we're sure there are still plenty of sexy adventures ahead of us!

6

JEALOUSY: AN OPPORTUNITY FOR INTIMACY AND PASSION (SERIOUSLY!)

Jealousy: Derived from the Old French word *gelos*, meaning "possessive and suspicious." Later modified with the suffix *lousy* to better describe what being in this emotional state feels like.

Yeah, we're kidding. But if you've ever been afflicted by this distressing and often debilitating emotion, as most of us have at one time or another, it sounds plausible, doesn't it?

I (Mali) should know. There was a time in my life when jealousy could take me over in an instant and have me behaving in ways that were very unpleasant.

One incident stands out in particular. I was attending a small university in the Appalachians and working part-time in the local family-owned hardware store. One Saturday I looked up from the register to see my boyfriend coming into the store. Ron, who I'd been dating about three months, wanted to purchase a pane of glass to replace a cracked window in his kitchen. I cut the glass on the big machine in the back of the store and we carefully placed it in his truck. With a kiss that promised more later, he was gone. I spent the rest of the afternoon daydreaming about our date that evening.

After work, I drove the winding mountain roads to his cabin, window rolled down, singing along with the pop songs blasting from the radio. Ten miles of hills and I was finally making my way up his rocky, makeshift driveway. Ron had just finished caulking around the new glass and looked quite pleased with the results.

We stepped into the kitchen to admire the view from the inside. He put his arm around me and said he had a surprise. A good friend had stopped by and given him two front-row tickets to the John Denver concert that evening.

I, however, was unimpressed and had no interest in going. At the time, I had no appreciation for country music or anything close to it. We got into a disagreement, me upset that he'd made plans without asking me, Ron frustrated that I wouldn't even consider going to see this living legend with him.

At some point in our exchange, Ron announced, "I'll have to leave soon to make it to the concert. I think I'll call Debbie and see if she wants to go. She's a huge Denver fan."

Debbie? His ex-girlfriend? On *our* date night? In a big, dramatic gesture, I slammed my fist right through the window he'd spent all afternoon installing. Glass and blood flew in every direction.

Ron rushed me to the sink and ran water over my hand. Despite his irritation over the broken window and my outburst, and his eagerness to get on the road, he was still a Southern gentleman. As he began to extract slivers of glass from my flesh, a wave of embarrassment at my angry reaction came over me, compounding the jealousy I was already feeling.

It was then I caught sight of the list of phone numbers taped to the side of his refrigerator. There she was: *Debbie*. The anger roared up again. I memorized her number.

After Ron had bandaged my cuts, I curtly told him to have a good time and took off. I drove down the hill, found a payphone, and dialed Debbie's number. I explained who I was. Although she had just gotten off the phone with Ron and was about to leave, she listened to what I had to say. She agreed that Ron calling her when I had a date with him was insensitive. Debbie sounded hesitant about her decision to meet up with him, and I found myself inviting her to skip the concert and join me for a drink instead. To my surprise, she said yes. I was curious to meet her—and secretly pleased that I had messed with Ron's plans for the evening.

Debbie was funny and easygoing, definitely someone I could have been friends with. As she talked about her friendship with Ron, especially their shared love of live music, I began to feel bad that I'd kept her from seeing the show. It occurred to me that Ron's assumption that I'd be thrilled by his surprise was understandable. From his perspective, this was a wonderful gift he had to give me. Unfortunately for both of us, it was one I wouldn't have appreciated until years later.

Somehow Ron and I got past this incident and dated for a while longer. It took me some time, but Ron, I eventually realized, hadn't been the cause of my jealous reaction. Instead, it stemmed from my belief that it wasn't right for a guy I was dating to spend time with another woman. This was a belief I'd picked up, along with many others, from my only relationship teachers at the time: family, friends, television, and movies.

Every time I've heard *Take Me Home, Country Roads* in the years since, I've felt a twinge of regret. If my ideas about love, dating, and music had been more mature at the time, I wouldn't have cheated myself out of the opportunity to see this American icon in person.

RATIONAL VS. IRRATIONAL JEALOUSY

Mali's story is about what we like to call irrational jealousy. Most instances of jealousy in romantic relationships are similar to this one, arising from our own insecurities and fears rather than from an actual break in trust. In other words, the source of this type of jealousy is something going on in our own mind rather than something actually happening out there. This is a crucial distinction. When the cause is dishonesty or actual infidelity, we experience what we call rational as opposed to irrational jealousy. Rational jealousy is based on fact rather than fiction.

I (Joe) have had personal experience with rational jealousy. I spent many years in a relationship that, at least for a while, I presumed to be monogamous. Presumed—until the day I returned home from an exhausting overseas work trip.

My partner's young son Keenan met me at the door. He was as excited to see me as I was to see him. Keenan chatted on about all the things that had happened while I was out of town. Then he burst out, "And Mike the Mailman came over for a visit!"

The heat rushed to my face. My stomach clenched into a knot.

"When was that?" I asked, trying to sound casual.

"Last *night*!" He hopped up and down with each word. "I was supposed to be *sleeping*!"

Keenan loved Mike the Mailman. Every afternoon he stared out the window in anticipation of the mail delivery. He and his mother often went outside to chat with Mike about his job.

"Why was Mike the Mailman here?"

"He had to deliver a special *package*!" Hop hop hop.

His innocent answers made the obvious even more obvious. I was devastated. Knowing that my girlfriend had been unfaithful was a terrible blow to my self-esteem. What I didn't know then is that this would turn out to be just the first of many such incidents.

Over the next couple of years, I learned firsthand that the Old French knew exactly what they were talking about with their word *gelos*. I became suspicious and possessive, always worried that someone else was getting my girlfriend's attention. My jealousy was at times all-consuming. It was hard to focus on anything else. *Where is she right now? Who is she talking to? What are they doing together?* There was a time when I looked with suspicion at almost every male she came into contact with. *Could it be him—is he next? Is she flirting with him? Have they slept together?*

Each time I had my suspicions confirmed and discovered that she was seeing yet another man, I felt angry and embarrassed all over again. I was carrying a deep sense of shame because I believed I couldn't satisfy her enough to keep her from having affairs.

I didn't want to break up. I liked our life together, and I loved being a stepdad to her son. So instead, I tried everything I could to get her to change. Each time it happened, I would threaten to leave if she didn't stop having affairs, eventually eliciting a promise from her that she would never do it again. As things settled down, I'd try to convince myself that this time she'd keep her promise and we could focus on the parts of our lives together that we enjoyed: the home we shared, our friends, and Keenan.

Now, my story is relatively extreme, involving not just imagined infidelity but actual infidelity, which is much more emotionally complex. The jealousy I experienced was mixed up with anger, disappointment, and feelings of shame and betrayal. I learned firsthand that actual infidelity creates more imagined infidelity. My tormented imagination was working overtime! Infidelity can also leave behind fears and insecurities that, even if you've moved on and are with a new partner, can take years to recover from.

If you've been cheated on, you may have personal experience with this. If you're still in that relationship or the subsequent healing process, you may want to jump to "And If the Threat Is Real?" later in this chapter. It's definitely okay to skip the rest of this chapter if you find the information triggering or unrelatable.

Irrational jealousy, which is not in response to an actual break in trust—the kind of jealousy in Mali's case—can be severely damaging to a relationship if left unchecked. Some people's jealousy is extreme, manifesting as controlling behavior, abuse, or violence. But even milder cases can end up being toxic to a relationship. The strain caused by even a low level of suspicion and unwarranted mistrust can lead to arguments, hurt feelings, and resentment and result in a partner pulling away or even a relationship's eventual demise. This kind of jealousy is the primary focus of this chapter.

Platonic Friendships

Let's look at one common area where irrational jealousy can be detrimental to a relationship: when one's partner has a platonic friendship with someone else. A platonic friendship is one that is nonromantic and nonsexual but may still involve feelings of love and affection. This could be a person someone shares an interest or hobby with, an old friend, or even someone they used to date. To feel fulfilled, everyone needs a variety of healthy relationships in their lives. Yet some people will try to prevent their partner from maintaining certain friendships—especially friendships with people of a particular gender—because of their own jealousy issues.

Lisa, a writer, says the relationship with her now–ex-husband deteriorated primarily because he insisted that she give up her close friendship with her childhood "bestie" solely because he was male. It took her three years to realize that she'd been so committed to making her marriage work that she had allowed her husband to control who she spent time with and who she didn't, and that the isolation had made her seriously depressed. One of the happiest days of her life, Lisa says, was reconnecting with that friend after leaving her husband. "I'll never clip my wings again to appease someone else's fears," she says.

Tom has traded massages with a friend ever since they were certified together several years ago. This type of exchange is a common practice among massage therapists. Tom chose to end a relationship with a woman who continually insisted he shouldn't be receiving massages from a female friend. His new wife Evelyn is not at all worried about the arrangement. "If something was going to happen, it would have happened way before I came into the picture!" Evelyn says.

Because of an experience similar to Lisa's and Tom's, Anita let her new boyfriend William know from the start that she performs acroyoga, an intensely physical form of partner yoga, with a male training partner. Anita and Aaron travel to several events a year, often sharing a hotel room to save on expenses. "I told William that I don't plan to stop performing with Aaron. However, I'll always answer any questions he has and will be available to reassure him. He's also welcome to come on our trips if he'd like to. But I won't give up this passion of mine just because he feels jealous or insecure." William says that he does occasionally feel nervous when Anita and Aaron are traveling, but knowing that he can call Anita at any time allows him to manage his nervousness. He also says he's learned to "enjoy the bittersweet feeling of simultaneously missing her and wanting her."

From Jealousy to Passion

Jealousy can hold couples back from exploring sexually, so understanding how it operates and having skills to work with it is immensely valuable. We'd also like you to consider the possibility that once you get a handle on this emotion, you might discover that a tinge of jealousy can actually be used to infuse your relationship with passion and excitement.

We understand that you might react to this statement with suspicion or downright disbelief. If so, we invite you to entertain the idea that, for some couples, a touch of jealousy, properly approached and channeled, can be an opportunity for intimacy and personal growth, as well as for firing up their desire.

For example, Candice is an avid tango dancer. "It's just the way it is that you go to these dances and play with each other's energy," she explains. "It's a sensual activity, and I always come home really turned on and ready to play!" But her previous boyfriend became upset every time she went dancing, accusing her of leading men on and wanting to have sex with them. Not only did he make Candice feel bad for something she was passionate about, but any sexual energy she might have brought home with her was completely wasted. His jealousy was so intense that Candice finally broke up with him. Her new boyfriend also feels a little bit jealous when she goes out, but he understands and accepts her love for tango. In addition, Candice says, "He very much appreciates the fact that I'm going to be horny for *him* when I get home!"

When Keisha's girlfriend has lunch with an ex-lover, Keisha likes the flashes of jealousy she experiences during that time. "I enjoy picturing her being her sexy, clever self with someone else who appreciates her!"

When Samuel's wife Kathleen goes out with her friends, he likes the little "jealousy high" it creates in him. He even helps her choose what to wear. "Then I'm at home thinking, 'She's so sexy in those skintight jeans!'" Samuel has always asked Kathleen "to tell me anytime she gets hit on, because I love hearing about any attention she gets." While she's out, Kathleen will tease him with a text: "I think the drummer's flirting with me!" A few sexy texts back and forth, and they both know they're going to have a good time that night.

For us, it's taken vulnerability, experimentation, and lots of heart-to-heart talks over the years to arrive at a point where we both *want* to feel a little jealous from time to time. We know from experience that an occasional visit from the green-eyed monster will get that rush going and instantly reconnect us with our desire and gratitude for each other. It also motivates us to do whatever we can to keep this great thing we have going!

Before we explore this idea in more depth, let's take a little side trip and talk about cheating. More specifically, let's talk about what cheating is *not*—and the strong link between imagined cheating and irrational jealousy.

Cheating: It's Not What You Think

When asked to give a definition of cheating, a common reply is, "Everyone knows what cheating is—having sex with someone else!" Yes, if two people have agreed to be monogamous and one has sex outside the relationship, that's clearly cheating. Estimates vary widely, but a substantial percentage of marriages are touched by this, what we could call "conventional cheating."

Beyond this, the question of what might constitute cheating can be more complicated. What about kissing—is that cheating? Many people would say yes, while others would say it depends on the type or length of the kiss. Some people would include romance in their definition of cheating: "Sexually or romantically engaging with someone else without your partner's knowledge or consent." An emotional affair, when a person is spending considerable time and attention on someone other than their partner, might fall under this definition, as could some online flirtations.

For a portion of the population, a wide variety of common activities count as cheating, from fantasizing to watching pornography to having close friends of a particular gender. People whose partners define such things as cheating often find themselves feeling frustrated and resentful.

We suggest these three guidelines for determining whether something is or isn't cheating:

1. **It's not cheating if it's just in their head.** If your position is that fantasizing about someone else is "mental infidelity," you're going to get cheated on regularly! Trying to regulate what's going on in someone else's head is just going to frustrate you both, and is bound to fail. The reality is, we can't even control what's going on in our *own* heads most of the time. And sexually fantasizing

about other people ranks among the top common sexual behaviors. In a study of 70,000 people in relationships, 61 percent of women and 90 percent of men reported having sexual fantasies about people they meet. The study found no correlation between such fantasies and how happy people felt in their relationships.[1]

2. **It takes two people to cheat.** It's not possible to cheat alone. Cheating requires two (at least!). This means that neither masturbating nor watching pornography are cheating. Along with fantasizing, these activities fall into the "zone of erotic autonomy" that author and sex-advice columnist Dan Savage wisely points out that all people, in a relationship or not, are entitled to. That said, compulsive or excessive masturbation or porn consumption can certainly be a problem if it's causing someone to neglect their responsibilities or their intimacy with their partner. Similarly, while noticing other attractive people isn't a betrayal of one's partner, gawking or blatantly staring at them is insensitive and disrespectful to their partner and, potentially, to the person they're staring at.

3. **It's not cheating just because it triggers your insecurities.** Some people assign the cheating label to things like chatting with an ex, having a celebrity crush, paying "too much" attention to the cheerleaders, or liking certain images on someone else's social media account.

Obviously, there's a lot of real cheating going on. And anyone who's faced actual infidelity knows how excruciatingly painful and difficult that can be. However, imagined cheating can have its own detrimental effects. It's challenging to have a truly connected relationship when one person feels they must constantly police the other's actions.

If you feel the urge to control your partner's behavior, take a deeper look at why. Are you defining these common behaviors as inappropriate or off limits in an effort to manage your own fears or insecurities? Or has your partner actually been dishonest or unfaithful? And if you're the person who is engaging in a behavior that your partner is frustrated over, be honest with yourself. *Is* there a reason for your partner to be concerned? *Are* they getting less of your attention? *Are* you being compulsive or dishonest? What's the motivation behind your behavior?

Rather than arguing about whether a particular behavior should be considered cheating or not, what's much more helpful is to see your difference of opinion as a sign that what's really needed are conversations to discover any fears, insecurities, or expectations underlying your conflicting ideas. If the two of you find it impossible to have honest, considerate conversations—rather than arguments—about your different perspectives, this is an area where the help of a neutral third party could be invaluable.

What are the benefits of not defining such things as fantasizing, watching erotica, or appreciating someone else's attractiveness as cheating? Even when we're fully committed to our partner and we do our best to keep our sexual connection feeling vibrant and alive, we may still enjoy the feeling of variety and autonomy that these common behaviors can offer us. When engaged in respectfully and thoughtfully, they can contribute sexual energy to the relationship and actually help some of us to stay happily committed. We'll circle back to this idea later when we explore the "just enough jealousy" edge.

TAKING CHARGE OF JEALOUSY

Almost universally, we don't like to admit when we're feeling jealous and we don't like how we feel and act when we are jealous. And most of us don't have effective ways of handling it. In many relationships where jealousy is an issue, one person is considerably more affected by it than the other, making things feel out of balance. For some people, for example, the mere mention of their partner's ex provokes strong feelings of jealousy, while for others it takes seeing their partner interact with someone they're obviously attracted to for jealousy to show up.

When jealousy comes on, it can be an emotional and physiological avalanche. Rather than being just a single emotion, the experience we call jealousy often involves a multitude of emotions, including fear, envy, anger, and sadness, as well as their related physiological effects, such as elevated blood pressure and heart rate.

If you or your partner struggles with jealousy, it helps to remember that these feelings are normal. Some experts think they may be an evolutionary instinct, nature's way of helping us protect what we have. Whether this emotion is evolutionary or not, most of us have been conditioned to believe that love and affection are limited commodities. This one idea is the cause of immeasurable suffering. If our partner shows interest in someone else, we've been trained to believe we will—and even should—react with jealousy. Even if their attention is only momentarily turned toward another, many of us have learned to interpret that as a loss of interest in us.

We've also been taught that reacting with jealousy will help us protect our interests. Yet those reactions are very often the cause of relationship conflict, rather than a solution. As we try to control certain situations or attempt to rein in our partner's behavior, frustration and resentment can build up on both sides. The more suspicious we are or the more control we try to exert, the more our partner is apt to pull away from us.

In circumstances where our jealousy is in response to a perceived threat to a relationship, not a real one, we're not experiencing jealousy because of what someone else is doing or might do. We're experiencing jealousy because of what we *tell ourselves* about what they're doing or might do.

Suppose your partner is at a party and enjoying a conversation with someone they find attractive and you're not there to witness it. Would the mere fact that they're having this interaction *cause* you to feel one way or another? Of course not. Now suppose you arrive at the party and see them engaged in this conversation. Any emotions that arise in you aren't caused by what your partner is doing. They are caused by what you believe or tell yourself about what they're doing.

Again, the focus here is on situations involving an imagined threat to a relationship, as in Mali's story of the John Denver concert tickets. If there's a solid reason to believe there might be a real threat—like the infidelity I (Joe) faced, or if your partner is manipulative, deceitful, or consistently ignores you while lavishing attention on others—jealousy would certainly be an understandable response. We cover situations like these in the section "And If the Threat Is Real?"

In addition, if you've had a traumatic experience with a previous partner, as Joe did, situations with your current partner that remind you of that trauma can trigger emotional and even physical symptoms. We talk more about this in the section "Transcending Jealousy—Together."

Jealousy can also be an automatic response to underlying beliefs about our inferiority or inadequacy, which might prompt thoughts like, "My partner is attracted to them because they're in such good shape" or "I just know I don't satisfy her." Jealousy can also be kindled by thoughts of comparison, like, "They're younger, hotter, sexier, more talented, more interesting than I am." Thoughts like these make us feel threatened, even when rationally we know we're not. We may believe that if we were "enough"—good enough, attractive enough, sexy enough, successful enough, muscular enough, endowed with large or small enough body parts—our partner wouldn't want anyone else. Jealousy-producing thoughts and beliefs may also involve the imagined loss of a lover's affection or a fear of being ignored or abandoned: "If he gets to know her, he'll wish he wasn't already committed to me." "She's bound to meet someone more confident and successful if she attends that motivational seminar."

Jealousy is sometimes a reflection of what isn't happening in our own relationship. For example, we might feel disappointed or insecure if our partner is showing someone else affection or attention when our own relationship could use some tending to.

In the midst of a jealous reaction, most of us have an impulse to blame our partner. In one way or another, we communicate this message: "My jealousy is your fault. You have to stop doing what you're doing, because I'm being hurt by it." Again, this reaction is often just what we've been taught.

When jealousy takes over, it's typically what's going on in our own mind, not someone else's behavior, that's the real source of our distress. By recognizing the true cause of our feelings and letting go of holding others responsible for our emotional state, we gain the ability to create a more positive experience for ourselves, whatever the circumstances.

Even if jealousy has been something you've struggled with in the past, it really is possible to make changes that will eventually have you feeling confident in your ability to approach jealousy in an empowered way in the future.

Self-Inquiry: Jealousy and You

When jealousy strikes, it can be like a temporary insanity, making it difficult to think clearly or act rationally. Because of this, if you're prone to jealousy, it's best to prepare yourself ahead of time.

An honest self-assessment will help you develop more awareness of where your jealousy comes from and how it affects you. So let's take a look at your personal history with jealousy: how you acquired it, what brings it on, what you tell yourself at those times, and what you've said and done while under its influence.

Take your time with these questions. Writing your responses down will help you think through these topics more thoroughly. Sharing your reflections with a close friend—or your partner, if that's possible in your situation—can lead to even more insights.

Examine your conditioning. What messages do you remember taking in about jealousy when you were growing up? These might have come from your family and friends, shows you watched, or even song lyrics you listened to. For example, romance movies and novels often convey the fallacy that someone who's truly committed to us will never be attracted to anyone else, or at least will never show it. Our friends, in an effort to be helpful, may subtly or not-so-subtly reinforce the notion that we need to be constantly on guard for any signs that our lover's attention is being diverted elsewhere. By questioning the validity of the beliefs that were handed down to you, you start to interrupt the process that produces jealous emotions. You begin to "un-condition" yourself.

Review your past experiences. Bring to mind any significant moments or events in which you experienced jealousy. What do you remember about the circumstances? Who was there and what did you do? How did you feel, emotionally and physically? Try to recall what you were telling yourself at the time, anything from "This could be trouble" to "Is she attracted to them?" to "They're losing interest in me." Even if you can't recall anything specific, imagine what relevant beliefs or thoughts you might have had, as even they can be revealing. Now try to see any connections between your ideas about what was happening and your experience of this event. For example, focusing on a thought like, "They're losing interest in me" can make a person feel increasingly unsettled and insecure.

Assess your prior behavior. Make an honest evaluation of anything you've said or done when jealousy was in control. Have you felt uncomfortable when you've noticed your partner looking at someone else? If so, how have you responded to that discomfort? Some common reactions to feelings of jealousy include trying to manipulate or restrict one's partner or accusing them of not being committed. Even without grounds for suspicion, some people secretly monitor their partner for signs that something could be going on. They might search through their phone, internet history, purse, or jeans. They might question their motives or actions or ask for an accounting of their activities. If their partner responds to these behaviors defensively, they might interpret that reaction as a sign that their suspicions are warranted. In reality, it could be that their partner has done nothing at all and just resents having their integrity questioned.

Examine the effects jealousy has had on you. Take a close look at any consequences your own jealousy has had on your life and relationships. Has it made you anxious, stressed, or depressed? Has it caused you to miss out on certain activities or friendships? In what ways has it affected your experiences with your partners? Has it caused you to lash out, break down, or withdraw? Have you had a relationship end because of jealousy?

Know your triggers. Identify the kinds of situations that commonly trigger a jealous reaction in you. Do you feel jealous when your partner is traveling or involved in events and activities that don't include you? How about when you're in the presence of certain people, such as someone who always seems happy to see your partner but not as interested in you? Or is jealousy more common for you if you're attending a social event and, for whatever reason, are not feeling at your best? Knowing your triggers is not necessarily so you can avoid these situations, but so you can bring more awareness to them and be prepared to work with jealousy if it does come up.

Thinking things through ahead of time will give you insight and perspective to help you defuse your reactions before they begin. For example, before going into a situation that's triggered your jealousy in the past, you might give yourself a pre-jealousy pep talk. That could sound something like this: "There will be attractive people at this party. So that I won't indulge in thoughts like 'I'm not attractive or interesting enough,' I'm going to put my full attention on whatever I'm doing. If I'm dancing, I'll focus on the music and the movement of my body. If I'm talking with someone, I'll put all my attention on our conversation. And if I'm feeling lonely, I'll go *find* someone interesting to talk to!"

What to Do in the Moment

Now that you have a better understanding of your personal history with jealousy and its effects on you, you'll be ready the next time it tries to take you over. Here's what to do when you start heading down the jealousy rabbit hole.

Cut yourself some slack. When you feel jealousy coming on, rather than criticizing or blaming yourself ("I shouldn't be reacting this way, this isn't who I want to be"), which is unhelpful and self-defeating, give yourself permission to feel what you're feeling. Underneath the jealousy there may be fear, anxiety, anger, or a lack of self-worth. Have some compassion. This isn't easy stuff!

Allowing yourself to feel what you're feeling and treating yourself with kindness will help you move through these powerful emotions and gain insight. Remember that jealousy is normal. Almost everyone feels it at one time or another, and you've been conditioned to experience it in certain situations. (This was certainly true for me, Mali, in the window incident. I had no idea I would react so violently to the thought of my boyfriend getting together with a former girlfriend.) Finally, remind yourself that you now have ways to work with these feelings and that things are going to be okay.

Don't let jealousy control your words or actions. It's almost always true that the longer you can do nothing in response to an onset of jealousy, the better off you will be. If you've manipulated people or situations in an attempt to alleviate your jealousy, learn how to stop this powerful emotion from controlling what you say or do. This takes awareness and practice, but it really is possible to train yourself not to let jealousy direct your words or actions.

Not allowing jealousy to control your behavior means resisting the urge to manipulate your partner or the situation and refraining from making sarcastic or accusatory comments. You might give yourself a time-out, like listening to some music or going for a short walk. This pause gives you the opportunity to examine where your reaction is coming from and take any actions or make any decisions from a more grounded, more aware place. You might even let your partner know that you're giving yourself some time and space to work with what's come up for you. And if you do let jealousy get the better of you for a while, try smiling and acknowledging that: "You got me this time, but next time I'll be ready for you!"

Examine the thoughts and beliefs underlying your feelings. At this point, you'll be able to take a look at the origins of your jealous feelings. If the threat is real rather than imagined—for example, if you've just discovered that your partner is having an affair—see the next section, "And If the Threat Is Real?" Otherwise, try to recall any relevant thoughts you were having at the time.

Make the connection between what you were thinking ("They've noticed that hottie over there. Now I'll get less of their attention" or "They're dressed so well. I feel totally outclassed") and how you subsequently feel (anxious, insecure, undesirable). Or try to identify an underlying belief or idea that could be activating your jealous emotions. Since jealousy is often a manifestation of our self-esteem issues, this underlying idea may be some version of "I'm not enough" (whether that's good enough, attractive enough, sexy enough, successful enough, and so on). Or it could be something like, "There isn't enough love for me" or "I don't belong" or "I'm unlovable." Write down any underlying ideas or beliefs you uncover. This will give you distance from those thoughts so you can assess them more objectively.

Imagine how you would feel without those thoughts or beliefs. As soon as possible after you've identified the thoughts or beliefs underlying your jealous feelings, take some time to imagine how your experience would be different if you were free from their influence. Picture yourself in the same circumstances, but without these ideas running through your mind. How would your experience play out? How would you feel? This exercise can give you insights you might use to guide your behavior in similar circumstances in the future. You might also discover that underlying the jealousy is something about you or your relationship that needs attention. For example, "I'm still having issues with trust since I was with so-and-so—maybe I should talk to someone" or "I'm not usually this insecure—is there something I need to ask for or communicate?" or "We've been distant lately. Is there something we or I can do to feel more connected?"

Trade up. Once you've identified a particular thought or idea that causes you to feel bad, it's sometimes possible to simply stop thinking that thought. Often though, because of years of conditioning and habitual thought patterns, you can't easily let go of a negative thought. You can, however, refocus your attention on a thought that makes you feel good instead. An effective replacement thought is not something you *wish* were true. It's an idea you accept *as* true. For example, if your thought was "I'm not attractive enough," you might recognize that the thought "I'm attractive in my own way, with many appealing qualities" is actually more accurate. Or instead of, "There are lots of interesting people at this party. I better keep an eye on my partner," try thinking, "There are lots of interesting people here. I'll have fun getting to know some of them."

Maintaining the self-awareness necessary for these practices can take substantial willpower. But when you consider the destructive potential of jealousy, it's well worth the effort.

Even if jealousy does succeed in getting the best of you for a time, you can come back to these ideas after things have simmered down. Look back over the incident and ask yourself, *What happened there? Why did I react that way? What was I telling myself and how did that make me feel? How would I have felt if I hadn't told myself those things?* If you said or did something you regret, you might share with your partner, and perhaps any other people involved, what was happening for you and what you're doing to undo those old patterns. This requires courage and vulnerability, but you might be surprised just how understanding others can be.

Finally, remember to be generous with the self-compassion. Feelings of shame can often prevent us from honestly looking at our own behaviors, thoughts, and beliefs. Admitting our feelings of inadequacy and insecurity, even just to ourselves, can be exceptionally challenging. Acknowledge yourself for your willingness to try, and forgive yourself if you don't make all the progress you'd like—this time. You might as well. Life being the way it is, there will always be a next time!

And If the Threat Is Real?

What if your partner is actually pursuing someone else behind your back or comes home and admits they're having an affair? Such situations are complicated by issues far beyond just jealousy. First, and most potentially damaging to the relationship, is the sense of betrayal you'll feel. If your partner has been physically intimate with someone else, there might be health consequences. And if their disclosure has you considering altering or even ending your relationship, that prospect could create instability or upheaval in your life. It would certainly affect any children who are involved and might also have substantial financial consequences.

In such a situation, you'll probably experience a range of intense emotions, jealousy being just one of them. Feelings of abandonment and low self-esteem will likely be in the mix as well. To make things worse, you may be amplifying those (quite valid) emotions by indulging in thoughts like, "How could they have done this to me after all we've been through? Don't I matter to them? They said they loved me!" A healthier approach can be to acknowledge the feelings you're experiencing, but to then make an effort to notice when you're intensifying those emotions through unproductive or obsessive thinking. This takes determination, to be sure, but is far more effective than allowing your thoughts and emotions to continually spiral out of control. You might also try various techniques for releasing painful emotions, such as meditation, mindfulness practices, acupuncture-point tapping techniques, hypnotherapy, or visualization, to find what works for you. Physical activities, from yoga and tai chi to hiking to pounding a punching bag or a pillow, can also help you release feelings of anger, frustration, and sadness in a healthy way. And of course, getting the perspective of someone you trust can be invaluable.

Do your best not to respond to the situation or make decisions out of feelings like anger, betrayal, or despair. Actions fueled by these emotions won't be guided by either wisdom or love. Before deciding how to move forward, get some perspective by talking things through with a close friend or counselor. Allow yourself the time necessary to make any decisions from a place of awareness and acceptance. Remember, accepting another's actions doesn't mean you approve of or condone them. Accepting is just acknowledging that this is how they are choosing to act right now. This acknowledgment can give you a clearer perspective on the situation.

I (Joe) learned firsthand about the transformative power of acceptance in my relationship with my unfaithful partner. Each time I discovered that she was having yet another affair, I'd get frustrated and angry and coerce her into promising never to do it again. The last time, though, was different.

It was a picture-perfect fall morning and I'd come upstairs to ask her a question. She was in her office talking on the phone. The door was closed. A feeling of dread welled up inside me. She never closed that door. Her voice was animated. She was laughing. And then came five words I can still hear clearly in my mind today: "And the sex is great!"

There was one thing I knew for sure. She wasn't talking about us!

I opened her office door with a heavy heart, bracing myself for the all-too-familiar confrontation to come. But there was nothing familiar about what occurred then.

She put down the phone, looked up at me, and announced, "You're not making me give this one up. I'm keeping this. I'm keeping this relationship."

I stood in the doorway, stunned. She wasn't following the pattern we'd established over the years and I had no idea how to respond.

What happened next is a blur. I remember getting into my car, thinking I'd drive the hour or so to the ocean and try to figure out what to do next. Or maybe I'd just keep going.

But somewhere between home and the coast, a realization dawned on me. Resisting who she was, which is what I'd done every time before, was never going to work. In that moment, I knew what I needed to do. I needed to accept that, for now, this was simply what she was doing and that she wasn't ready to change.

A huge wave of relief moved through me.

I turned the car around. Every tree I passed on the drive back home glowed in the soft fall light. It really was a beautiful day. I loved living here.

Back home, I walked into her office and told her it was okay, that I understood. She seemed relieved, but nervous. I wasn't playing out the role of "distraught, angry boyfriend" that she'd come to expect.

I spent the rest of the afternoon in a state of peaceful serenity. Looking back, I can see now that in the very moment that I accepted who she was, my life changed forever. All the jealousy, shame, anxiety, and anger that had weighed me down for years simply evaporated. Incredibly, it was my acceptance of who she was that enabled me to finally move on from that unhealthy, unfulfilling relationship.

What I discovered that day is that even in a situation involving actual betrayal or infidelity, much of our suffering comes from what we tell ourselves it all means. This can be a challenging concept to grasp. But it wasn't my girlfriend's *behavior* that caused most of the pain I'd experienced, it was what I'd *told myself* her behavior meant. Her infidelities, I had believed, meant I wasn't good enough, attractive enough, or man enough. Today, I know that none of this was true. Her compulsion to have affairs, and her inability to be honest with me about them, stemmed entirely from her own insecurities and lack of self-esteem. They had nothing to do with whether or not I was good enough.

Leaving a partner who is continually unfaithful and isn't interested in or capable of changing is not usually the answer that people suffering in this kind of situation are looking for. They may spend months or years searching for just the right words, book, or therapy to magically change their partner into the person they wish they were. In such situations, it can be revolutionary to finally recognize that, for whatever reasons, their partner isn't going to change, and to consider that beginning the process of moving on may in fact be the best solution for everyone involved.

If this describes your situation, it's also important to know that you *can* survive, you *can* be happy, even if it means not having this person in your life in the same way. Getting support from people you trust and focusing on all the good that came from the relationship will help you immensely in finding your way through this transition.

On the other hand, if you're facing infidelity in your relationship and your partner *is* willing to address it, explore if there's any way to heal the damage that's been done and get to a more connected place. Darius, who is now in his fifties, left his wife when he discovered she'd been having an affair. His belief at the time, given to him courtesy of the society in which he'd grown up, was that infidelity equals divorce. It didn't occur to him that it might have been an opportunity for them to develop a deeper intimacy together. Years later, Darius says, after he and his ex-wife successfully co-parented from two separate households, he realized they might have been able to work through that difficult time, stay together with their two children, and even grow closer through that experience.

What If Your Partner Is Jealous?

Finally, what if you are dating or living with someone who is frequently jealous when you feel you've given them no cause to be?

It can be frustrating and exhausting to be the target of someone's unwarranted suspicions and have to constantly deny their accusations, reassure them, or deal with their possessive or controlling behavior. You've probably learned the hard way that pressuring them to change only results in more anger and resentment, for both of you.

First, do whatever you can to take care of yourself. When your partner points to you as the cause of their jealousy, just knowing that their feelings are their responsibility can give you some healthy distance from the situation. Talking to friends or family members can help you see your situation more objectively.

Second, understand that only the person who is experiencing the jealousy can ultimately overcome it. If they're not inclined to take responsibility for their behavior or make the effort to improve it, you have a choice to make. Leaving can be a very difficult decision, especially if there are children involved or you've been together a long time. Many people don't make this choice until they've spent a long time struggling to improve things. Yet the truth is that it's almost always the best choice for someone in an abusive or violent situation. And unwarranted jealousy often accompanies other unhealthy behaviors, like verbal, physical, financial, and sexual abuse. If your relationship has the potential for violence around jealousy or any other issue, make it a priority to find professional assistance or other support.

Third, remember that people who are irrationally jealous have low self-esteem. It's also often true that someone who stays with an irrationally jealous partner—especially if that partner isn't interested in doing what's necessary to address their jealousy—also suffers from low self-esteem. If you decide to change your level of involvement in the relationship or get out altogether (if you have children or are financially dependent, that can take time), use the opportunity to raise your own sense of self-worth. This will help you avoid attracting this dynamic into your life again.

Of course, this is all assuming that your partner's jealousy is in response to a *perceived* threat to your relationship, not an actual one. If your actions are posing a genuine threat, you've got some real soul searching to do! Spend some time honestly contemplating what you're doing and why you're doing it. You might want to reflect on questions like, *Is this the relationship I want to be in right now? And if it is, how do I want to treat my partner? What kind of person do I want to be?*

TRANSCENDING JEALOUSY—TOGETHER

Let's return to that very common type of jealousy in romantic relationships, the kind provoked by a person's own insecurities and fears rather than the kind stemming from an actual break in trust. Once a couple has an understanding of how this emotion operates, they might find it possible to help each other explore and address any jealousy that arises for either of them. In this way, jealousy can provide a unique opportunity for intimacy.

First, a point of safety. This is an advanced relationship practice that requires a strong, solid connection. If your partner is disinterested in, defensive about, or dismissive of talking about topics like jealousy, conversations like these might be impossible. And certainly if your relationship has the potential for physical, verbal, or emotional violence or abuse, the suggestions that follow are not intended for you. Instead, we recommend you get perspective on your situation and decide on the best course of action. Help is always available, whether that's professional support (often at low or no cost through county or city programs), friends, family, domestic abuse hotlines, or crisis text lines.

The ideas that follow also depend on the two of you having an established history of healthy communication. If you've had difficulties talking about complex or emotionally charged topics, work on your listening and communication skills first, perhaps with the help of a counselor, before moving ahead.

When you're both ready to try this process, the basic idea is simple. If it's your partner experiencing the jealousy, your role is to provide a calm, non-judgmental space for them to start looking at their reactions and get to the heart of what's causing them. Remembering that jealousy is often an indication of insecurities or limiting beliefs a person has about themselves, you can help your partner consider the thoughts and ideas behind their reactions and how those thoughts or ideas are making them feel.

It can take tremendous courage to share jealous feelings and thoughts, so give your partner your full attention and listen compassionately. Imagine yourself in their place and try to understand things from their point of view. If it feels appropriate, offer reassurance, such as that you love them, are still deeply attracted to them, and are very happy with the relationship you have. When your partner seems receptive, you might also share your own perspective on the situation. Then, together, come up with some replacement thoughts for them to try out the next time jealousy surfaces.

For example, I (Mali) have a lifelong history of making negative mental comparisons between myself and others, such as, "She's so much more stylish than I am" or "She's younger than me, I look old next to her." This type of habitual thought pattern is often set in motion, and continually reinforced, by the families and societies in which we live. Our negative comparisons become negative perceptions, giving us a skewed version of reality and of ourselves. With the work I've done on my own insecurities and jealousies over the years, those voices have grown much quieter. When they do surface, it's so helpful to have Joe's reassurance and willing assistance with examining and letting go of my negative comparisons and perceptions.

Joe and I have an open invitation to reach out to each other for help with this kind of mental reprogramming. Together we can take a look at the direct link between what I'm telling myself (that I'm not stylish enough, young enough, and so on) and how I subsequently feel (usually terrible!) and come up with alternative ideas that will support me rather than make me feel "less than." It's often easier for someone else—whether that's a partner, a friend, or an experienced counselor—to come up with replacement thoughts for us, as they're in a position to be more objective. So in place of thinking, "I look too old next to her," Joe might suggest something like, "When I smile and am excited about life, it makes me look and feel younger" or "My beauty radiates from within" or "There is beauty to be appreciated at every age!" I try them out and hold tight to the ones that work for me.

Occasionally, a traumatic incident from the past that someone hasn't entirely worked through can produce residual feelings of jealousy and insecurity. Identifying and transforming these feelings and negative associations with the help of a loving partner can be tender and intimate and very beneficial for the relationship itself. Whenever we help our partner make a breakthrough with a challenging past event or current situation, our relationship expands in connection, safety, and depth.

I (Joe) can personally relate to this. After I met Mali, I would occasionally experience small emotional "aftershocks" from my previous girlfriend's infidelity. Any indication of Mali's attention being diverted elsewhere would feel like a little warning sign. If I saw her interacting with another man, a sense of uneasiness would come over me. Then there was the time I heard her on the phone with a male friend, with a closed door between us, and I was emotionally transported back to those days of suspicion and heartache. There was no rational reason for my reactions. They were just a reminder of a time when my girlfriend chatting up a new guy or talking in secret often meant trouble.

Mali has been highly sensitive to this. She was always willing to talk about what triggered me and reassure me. And she consistently demonstrates through her words and actions that our relationship is nothing like the one I was in previously. This has enabled me to create new and positive associations with what it means for my partner to interact with other men.

For just a moment, imagine that instead of dating Mali, I had started seeing someone else who, rather than being understanding about my emotional "aftershocks," was annoyed or dismissive. Suppose this hypothetical girlfriend had been talking with a male friend on the phone and noticed I was a little uneasy. Instead of taking the time to draw me out about what was coming up for me, imagine she said something like, "What, don't you trust me? Don't you know that we're good? There's nothing going on here!" Instead of becoming an opportunity for intimacy, it would have probably resulted in me shutting down emotionally. It certainly wouldn't have helped me heal from my previous relationship in the way that Mali's sensitivity and compassion have done.

Here's a similar story from clients we've worked with on their approach to jealousy.

Amanda and Jordan, a tech couple in their early thirties, have been married for three years. Although Amanda trusts Jordan implicitly, she still becomes insecure when they take yoga together and there's an attractive woman in class with them. She struggles to stay focused on what she's doing while tormenting herself with thoughts like, "Is Jordan watching her? She looks amazing in that pose. Is she trying to get his attention? Does he wish he could be with her instead of me?" Her inner monologue makes Amanda feel sullen and sad. Later, she sometimes can't stop herself from questioning Jordan about where his focus had been during class. These interactions are awkward and unnerving and by far the greatest source of conflict in their relationship.

"Here I have a husband who's devoted to me," Amanda says, "and I can see how my jealousy could cause enough stress between us to slowly drive us apart."

Because both Amanda and Jordan understand that he is not responsible for the thoughts she's having, he's able to stay in a neutral place and help her disentangle herself from them. When Amanda has a jealous reaction, she now waits until she's calmed herself down to initiate a conversation about it. She shares with Jordan the thoughts she had, the feelings she experienced, and any underlying ideas or beliefs she recognizes were affecting her.

"I can sure see the influence of my conditioning in my jealous thought patterns," Amanda says. "My thinking goes something like this: 'Jordan's looking at her and that's dangerous. If I were more attractive, more interesting, more whatever, he wouldn't be interested in her.' There's also this belief running in the background: 'Jordan shouldn't be attracted to anyone else. If he really loved me, he would only pay attention to me.'"

Amanda understands that her husband's perspective is likely to be more rational and trustworthy than her own on this issue, as his thinking isn't being influenced by insecurity and fear. So she's open to hearing his experience of the events. Knowing that, at its core, jealousy is about the fear of loss—whether that's the loss of love, attention, or one's partner—Jordan also takes this opportunity to reassure Amanda that she's not going to lose him.

"Yes, there are sometimes attractive women in class, and yes of course I notice them," he might tell her. "But mostly I'm just trying to keep my balance! And I'm completely attracted to *you*, totally in love with *you*. Another pretty woman won't suddenly make me want to give up what we have to try to go run off with her."

Over time, through these conversations, Amanda's self-defeating inner voice is calming down and has a lot less effect on her when it does start up. Even if that voice never goes away entirely, she now knows not to listen to everything it tells her as though it were "the truth." Both Jordan and Amanda say these intimate conversations not only bring them closer together, but are making yoga an activity they can now both look forward to.

This is most likely a very different kind of interaction than what's been modeled for you by families, friends, and every romantic comedy you've ever seen, so it might take some practice to get the hang of it. If you're both ready to try out this approach, start with a situation in which you feel only a small charge of jealousy. Share your thoughts in a no big deal, nonblaming way, along the lines of: "Here's what I was thinking.... Here's how those thoughts made me feel.... And here's why I might have learned to think this way...."

If your partner is working with jealousy, try to understand how, given their past and the thoughts they're having, they might end up with the feelings they have. Really do your best to put yourself in their place. Then, sharing your own perspective on the incident can often help your partner evaluate whether their fears are realistic (they rarely are!). As always, your empathy and reassurance will let them know they're being heard and understood. This will help calm their fears so that the two of you can get creative about how you might approach such a situation next time.

Remember that when you're working with deeply conditioned beliefs, you're unlikely to eliminate them all at once. If you keep at it, however, in time you *will* make progress.

"This process helps me quiet my irrational 'I'm going to lose him' response by evaluating how logical those thoughts actually are," says Amanda. "I can see that my fears are out of touch with reality. Jordan's not going to leave me for some random person he saw in yoga class. That's silly! But in the moment, my ability to logically assess what I'm telling myself is overwhelmed by the intensity of my emotional reaction. Giving myself time to reflect on what happened, and talking it through with Jordan later, helps a lot. And it's true: it does get easier over time."

THE "JUST ENOUGH JEALOUSY" EDGE

I (Mali) have done a lot of work on my jealousy since that afternoon I threw my fist through my boyfriend's kitchen window. Once I'd had time to reflect, it became clear that my jealousy hadn't been caused by anything Ron had done. Instead, it was created by the story I was telling myself, one I'd been conditioned to believe. That story went something like this: "It's disrespectful and dangerous for my boyfriend to be friends with, interact with, or even look at another woman." I didn't ever want to feel that crazy and out of control again. It was excruciating and humiliating. I became determined to rewire my attitudes and thought patterns.

By my mid-twenties, I was telling myself a very different story: "It's natural for my boyfriend to be friends with, interact with, and notice other women." This new story made all the difference. I felt empowered, no longer at the mercy of this emotion. In fact, when a man I was dating did the guilty eye-dart—spotting someone attractive when we were out together, then quickly looking off in another direction as if he hadn't seen what he'd just seen—I'd smile and say that I'd prefer he just look. The last thing I wanted, I'd explain, was for him to feel free to be himself only when he was alone or with friends and never when he was with me. Once past their initial skepticism, the men I've been in relationship with have found my attitude refreshing.

Before I go on, let me be very clear. I'm not talking about the kind of guy who would treat me disrespectfully, staring or gawking at women around us and ignoring me. I have zero tolerance for such behavior and would never date a guy who acts this way.

Telling myself this new story helped me to relax and have more fun too. It also led to a relationship-changing revelation: experiencing jealousy only rarely, and just a little at a time, can start to feel exciting instead of frightening.

And it *is* exciting—literally! The physiological state of arousal—characterized by increased heart rate, blood pressure, and so on—is the same state, whether the source is anger, jealousy, or sexual passion. What makes it feel different is its intensity and the meaning we give it.

Let's say Joe and I are working out at the gym. At some point, I notice him chatting with someone I know he finds attractive. When I feel that little flutter in my stomach, I could label it jealousy—and instantly feel fearful, suspicious, and just lousy overall. But if I instead say to myself, "Ooo, that's my desire for Joe getting stirred up there!" it feels a whole lot better. I feel excited and turned on. It makes me want him!

We're not the only couple who has learned to enjoy the state of arousal that's activated through a little jealous energy. Some couples who have been together a long time, for example, say they have no fear they will lose each other, so for them a little bit of jealousy feels safe to play with and can generate plenty of excitement.

That said, we can't emphasize enough that the ideas that follow are not for everyone. If you can't comprehend why anyone would ever want to do something to intentionally bring on a little jealousy, take that as a sign that these suggestions probably aren't for you. But even though these ideas may only be of interest to a small percentage of couples, that's still a very large number. So here goes!

Playing on the "Just Enough Jealousy" Edge

Once you've practiced using the tools for defusing and even preventing jealousy, you might be surprised to find that you actually *enjoy* feeling that rush of energy every once in a while. You will have discovered that instead of jealousy using you, you can use *it*. Properly channeled, jealousy can become an erotic fuel for charging up your sexual connection.

For example, a little jealousy can motivate you to make sure your relationship is as connected as possible. When I (Joe) see another guy checking Mali out, I feel that rush of energy that makes me check in with myself and ask, "Am I fully engaged in this relationship? Am I making sure to appreciate her? Am I doing everything I can to keep myself as happy, as healthy, and as hot as possible?" (And yes, I hope to still be asking myself that last one when I'm eighty!)

You can also teach yourself to convert a little jealous energy into excitement and desire. From a physiological perspective, you're taking advantage of the body's natural response to perceived danger. When you encounter something that your mind identifies as a potential threat, like a snarling dog or a romantic competitor, your bloodstream floods with "fight or flight" hormones and propels your body into a state of readiness. With practice, you can learn to reinterpret the heightened state of "just enough jealousy" as passion for your partner—and put it to good use.

For instance, for me (Mali), the idea that Joe might chat up someone attractive when he's out running errands can fire me up enough to seduce him the moment he walks back through the door. Or suppose I'm planning a trip out of town and imagine Joe turning our home into a bachelor pad for the weekend. The flutter of jealousy conjured up by these imaginings might inspire me to plan out a sexy evening for us before I leave, and another when I get back!

Jealousy also instills a sense of gratitude, as it helps us to tap into the fear of losing what we have. This loss isn't just a fear, but an eventual certainty. The truth is, we can only fully appreciate having someone in our lives when we completely grasp the reality that we could lose them in an instant, with no warning and no opportunity to say good-bye. Although we all know this on some level, most of us rarely give it any thought. A little jealousy can be a potent reminder of how much your relationship deserves to be cherished and how much you appreciate even the simplest things, like just getting to wake up together. Jealousy can help keep us from taking what we have together for granted.

Two people, of course, may have very different thresholds for what arouses just enough jealousy. Some people might feel intensely anxious when their partner just mentions the name of an ex-lover. For others, hearing about their partner's previous romantic relationships and sexual experiences is exciting. This is true for Dana: "I get to learn more about her, and in a very intimate way," Dana explains. "Besides, it's so hot to picture her being a wild thing back in college!"

For someone who's done a lot of work on their jealousy, or just naturally isn't the jealous type, it can take some effort to provoke a little of that possessiveness.

For instance, it used to be that whenever his wife went out with her friends, Wendell would sit at home growing more and more anxious. He knew that Angela could meet someone attractive while she was out. Even though he wasn't worried she would act on that, he still became insecure thinking about the possibility. These days, however, Wendell has become very good at monitoring what he's telling himself. He'll notice when he's thinking thoughts like, "This is bad, I have something to lose here" and talk himself into a better mindset, saying to himself, "She's not going home with anyone. She's going to come home feeling randy and ready to have sex with me!" This practice works well for him. Even a bit too well! He's realized that experiencing no nervousness when Angela goes out is not nearly as exciting. Now to activate a little of that feeling of uncertainty, Wendell will think back to things he used to say to himself, like, "Is she flirting with someone? She's wearing those skinny jeans. She's looking for attention! And she's got that cute friend with her. That could mean trouble." When Wendell takes this approach, he's almost always waiting up for Angela—with a smile on his face and the sheets turned down!

Teasing Out a Touch of Jealousy

If you're both ready, talk about where each of your edges are, while understanding that those edges can change in different circumstances and over time. What, right now, would get each of you to feel just a hint of jealousy?

For me (Joe), the answer to this question might be something like, "You talking to that handsome personal trainer just outside my line of sight!" We spend a lot of time at the pool and the gym, so there are plenty of opportunities for us to play with generating just enough jealousy. When I see Mali in conversation with another guy, say in the weight room, it puts me on high alert. I'll instantly compare myself to him, thinking, "What kind of shape is he in? How's my body compared to his? He's taller than I am, and he's got that dark hair that Mali really likes." Ideally, she will seem interested, but not *too* interested. Just interested enough to get me thinking about whether there's something for me to worry about and if it's time to step up my game! In contrast to earlier times when I would have compared myself unfavorably and felt insecure, I become motivated to be the best I can be. It's inspiring and empowering.

Have fun experimenting with creating situations that bring on just enough jealousy for each of you. You want to feel that nervousness in your chest and that tightening of your stomach, but not distressed or out of control. Trust us—a little bit of jealousy goes a long way!

Watching your partner interact from a distance can help you see them differently and reconnect with your attraction to them. Recently I (Mali) was sitting at a table at our favorite local music venue as Joe went up to the bar to order us drinks. While he was waiting to catch the bartender's eye, a beautiful woman struck up a conversation with him. Now, some people would feel threatened by this. They might even rush up to interject themselves into the conversation and bring the interaction to an end. Not me—I love the opportunity to be a voyeur of my guy! I actually stood up and moved a little off to the side so I could view Joe from the same perspective she was seeing him from. He seemed so sweet and friendly and, I must say, good-looking! Seeing him through her eyes sent a surge of appreciation and desire right through me.

A word of caution. Don't get caught up in the idea of "fairness," or the notion that what one of you is comfortable with, the other should be comfortable with too. You're two different people, with different experiences, desires, insecurities, and things to learn and unlearn. It will quite likely take more for one of you to feel a little flutter of jealousy than for the other to feel the same. "Fair" in this context means you play with your lover at their edge and they play with you at yours.

Leah's husband, for example, loves to hear fantasies she has about other men, and they both enjoy playing with them. "It makes for great foreplay!" she says. For Leah, though, listening to a fantasy

Danny might have about someone else is, at least for now, beyond her "just enough jealousy" threshold.

"I realize this sounds like a double standard," she explains. "But Danny knows there are things in my past that make this crazy difficult for me. He also knows I don't want it to be like this forever."

Her husband's understanding nature has allowed Leah to experiment a little around this. She's gone so far as to tell Danny a couple of stories she dreamt up about him and a fictitious college girlfriend he had. Because she's in control of the narrative, she can take the scenario right to the edge of her excitement—and not beyond. As Leah becomes more comfortable, she may decide to elaborate on their sexy storytelling sessions. She might even give Danny a suggestion for a story he could tell her.

In using the energy of jealousy to recharge your sexual connection, understand that if there were no risk, there would be no opportunity for excitement. So if you're learning how to play on that "just enough jealousy" edge, you or your partner might occasionally cross the line. (If you never do, you probably haven't gotten close enough!)

When you're there for each other, you can allow yourselves a little jealousy and know it will be okay. Remember to use empathy and reassurance generously. A reminder like, "I'm not going anywhere" or "We can stop anytime, you're in charge here" can make all the difference.

Designing a "Just Enough Jealousy" Adventure

If the two of you are ready, here are a few starter ideas for generating just enough jealousy.

If you've been in your relationship a while, it can be exciting to pretend that you're both single again, together. Walk through a market, along a boardwalk, or down a city street a little ways apart, imagining yourselves to be two single people. Who do you notice?

How do you feel? Get an impression of your partner as a free, autonomous spirit who's available to meet someone new. How does that feel? Are you able to stir up a little bit of jealousy? Check each other out, remembering that you are strangers and don't know each other's story. When you make eye contact, see if you can tap into that feeling of chemistry or sexual energy between you.

Take this "single again" suggestion a step further by walking into a club or party separately and observing each other interact. Remind yourself that it's safe and sexy when you know you're going home together. By watching your partner make a little friendly conversation with someone new, you might be able to provoke a touch of jealousy—just enough to compel you into seducing them to come home for some private playtime!

Here's another little adventure for the next time you're at a restaurant or party. Choose a comfortable vantage point where you can be close together while you observe the people around you. One at a time, take on the role of the "watcher" by letting your gaze move about the room naturally. Allow yourself to simply notice when someone catches your attention, just as you might if you were out by yourself or with friends. (Note that we said "notice" not "stare at.") Many of us have been taught that when we're with our partner, it's disrespectful to visibly find other people attractive. If you both think you're ready to let go of this notion and be more relaxed when you're out together, remember that it can take time and reassurance to unravel those years of conditioning.

When your partner is the watcher, focus your attention on their face. As they scan around the room, just be receptive. If someone catches their eye, you'll know it. You may even be able to feel what they're feeling. That little bit of "attraction energy" can even become something you're able to play with and enjoy together. In the process, you're turning a very common and potentially separating experience, one that many couples struggle with, into a uniquely connecting experience. You might also discover that encouraging your partner to feel at ease looking around a room in your presence, especially if they've had to monitor and restrict their gaze in previous relationships, will make them even more crazy about you.

By playing at your "just enough jealousy" edges together, you transform the energy of jealousy into appreciation and desire and effectively disarm one of the greatest relationship wreckers there is. Rather than being something to fear, jealousy becomes a catalyst for healing, creativity, and adventure, as well as for continually renewing your intimacy and your sexual connection.

I (Mali) would love to tell you about one of my favorite "just enough jealousy" adventures. One evening we were out at our local tapas bar, happy to have it all to ourselves. Then, within a span of about fifteen minutes, a series of men began arriving, one by one, until every stool was taken. We just had to ask these guys what was going on!

A couple of them confessed that they'd come for a singles' event but were too nervous to get off their stools and over to the banquet room where it was being held. So I said, loudly enough for them all to hear, "Hey Joe, why don't you go check it out for them?"

The entire row of men, including the bartender, looked stunned at my suggestion. Their expressions were easy to read: what woman in her right mind would send her guy into a room full of single women? They all watched as Joe shot me a smile, hopped off his stool, and strolled across the dining room to graciously fulfill his mission.

The woman at the entrance handed Joe a name tag and he started to mingle with the crowd. In less than a minute he had disappeared from our view, surrounded by women. Ah yes, here it came—that delicious feeling of just enough jealousy.

Obviously, this was a very contained and safe situation, as I knew he'd be right back. It was sexy to think of him being the center of all that feminine attention. I knew how much he'd enjoy it. Plus he'd have me to thank for the opportunity!

Eventually the woman in charge realized Joe wasn't actually single—she saw him pointing across to the bar and explaining his mission and where all the men were—and she asked him to leave. He came back wearing a big grin. Turns out he was the only man in the room. He gave the guys a quick pep talk: "You made it this far, you might as well take a chance! You just have to say hi and be friendly. A smile and hello goes a long way!"

Ten minutes later, we had the place to ourselves again.

HARNESSING THE ENERGY OF ATTRACTION

When we're really in love, our attraction to others does tend to lessen significantly. And some couples really do only have eyes for each other. But the majority of us don't suddenly stop being attracted to other people the moment we commit to a sexually exclusive relationship.

When asked, a lot of people say they would never be comfortable with the idea of their partner experiencing any degree of attraction to anyone else. There are valid reasons for feeling this way. We might be with someone we don't know that well yet—it takes time to build real trust. If we've experienced infidelity in the past, it can take even longer. Or perhaps we're with someone who has been dishonest, who has embarrassed us with rude or inconsiderate behavior, or who frequently disregards how we're feeling. And for some of us, our conditioning just runs too deep to feel we could ever change, and perhaps we don't even *want* to change.

All that said, it can be wonderfully freeing to let go of the jealousy and fear often associated with the thought that our partner might occasionally be attracted to someone other than us. What's more, when people who are committed to each other both believe that attractions to others are natural and healthy—and have enough self-awareness and compassion to talk about such things without judgment or fear of repercussions—they can use whatever erotic charge an outside attraction brings with it to keep the sexual energy between them activated. The openness and receptivity at the heart of these conversations creates even more intimacy, as true intimacy is about being authentic and vulnerable.

Vanessa and Robert have been happily monogamous for several years. They agree that it's unrealistic to expect that because they're committed to each other, they'll never again be attracted to anyone else.

"We think it's healthier to acknowledge when we find someone else attractive than to pretend it's not happening," Vanessa explains.

For Robert, freedom from the guilt of having attractions he's not "supposed" to have, and from the need to hide or repress those attractions, produces tremendous gratitude for Vanessa and the relationship they have.

"Here's this woman I'm so in love with, and we can talk about something that's usually verboten," he says. "That's exciting!"

Another couple, Addison and Cody, love to play a couple's version of the game "Who Would You Do?" They will sit close together in a café when they're on vacation, talking about what they each find attractive in the people who pass by. "Do you fancy them?" "Are they your type?" they'll whisper to each other. Eventually they return to their hotel room and enjoy all the sexual energy they've stirred up.

Kiran and Kristie play a similar game. On their date night, they'll leave their kids with the grandparents and go out to a nightclub. As they enjoy their drinks, they take their time looking around and choosing who they each might want to spend some alone time with if they were single again. Playing their secret game keeps them quite entertained and they go home erotically energized.

In another variation of this game, each person chooses someone they think is their partner's type. If you're up for trying this version, the outcome might surprise you. Kiran and Kristie were shocked the first time they played this way. They weren't even close to guessing each other's preferences!

Remember, ideas like these are for couples who are excited to try them. They may not be right for you or your partner—and that's perfectly okay.

Flirting: A Way to Play at Love

Let's talk about another way some couples use the energy of attraction to activate a little sexual energy and charge up their own relationship: by allowing themselves to occasionally interact with others in playful, mutually enjoyable ways. This could be as simple as momentarily catching someone's gaze and acknowledging each other's presence.

"That spontaneous expression of mutual attraction is very fulfilling," explains Karina, a married mother and teacher. "A few moments of receptive eye contact can energize my whole day!"

Valerie has been married for seven years and has twin toddlers. She had several relationships before settling down and always thought that being with just one person indefinitely would be difficult for her. Being flirtatious is her release.

"Just allowing myself to feel drawn to other people when I'm out running errands helps me feel very satisfied with my life," Valerie says. "You might think this would lead to an affair, but being able to express myself like this actually leads to more sex with my husband. And he's happy about that!"

There are both psychological and physiological reasons why a little healthy, safe flirtation can be beneficial for people in long-term relationships. Playfully interacting with someone we find interesting or attractive, and having that playfulness reciprocated, is an instant boost to our self-confidence. It's not that our partner's attraction to and appreciation of us isn't valuable—not at all. It's just nice to get that little reminder that we're still attractive to people who don't happen to be our partner. Flirting can also activate several of the "feel good" hormones, including dopamine, serotonin, oxytocin, endorphins, and even testosterone. In a strongly connected relationship, we can easily direct all of this stirred-up positive, playful energy right back into our relationship.

With flirting, like anything else, what we're comfortable with or feel is appropriate is often heavily influenced by our culture. Some people are raised in societies where even making eye contact is disapproved of, while others are much more at ease with physical attraction and even affection between nonlovers.

"When my friends all come together in a group," says Silvia, "maybe a third of them are single, everybody is affectionate, and there's no jealousy. We all enjoy being flirtatious, and we all understand it's not going anywhere. It's very Italian, very beautiful, very let's live life and enjoy."

As people often define flirting along the lines of "interacting with someone in order to have sex with them," it's no wonder many of us consider it off limits in a committed relationship. As Richard, who was recently married, puts it, "Flirting is for single people. Once you're in a relationship, it sends the wrong message." Richard has a valid concern. If there's a lack of understanding between a couple about what constitutes healthy, safe flirtation versus dangerous flirtation, flirting with someone else can communicate to your partner that they're not enough. In addition, it can indicate to the other person that you're available when you're not.

The kind of flirtation we're talking about here is not encouragement for anything to happen beyond that brief interaction. It's certainly not about promoting false hope in someone else.

With these ideas in mind, let's consider another definition of flirting, one right out of the dictionary: "A way to play at love." Approached like this, being flirtatious is simply allowing ourselves to interact in healthy, nonsexual ways with no purpose beyond feeling attractive and attracted. This is flirtation without any agenda or the need for any particular outcome. It's not about attempting to start something romantic or sexual. Instead, it's a simple, lighthearted "I see you" acknowledgment. This kind of flirtation—like exchanging an appreciative smile with a stranger—can be a healthy affirmation that we are still attractive and desirable.

"I'm a very flirtatious person; it's in my DNA," explains Gerise. "And in all these years selling men's clothing, I've had a lot of opportunities! To me, flirtation takes an ordinary interaction and makes it more enjoyable. You both feel better about yourselves when you've just left an interaction like this. To me, flirting is about *playing*, not *pursuing*."

Sydney, in her forties, feels the same way. "I need to be able to be my flirty, outrageous self wherever I am, and any guy who's boyfriend-worthy has to be evolved enough to know that my nature isn't a threat," she says. "And me flirting with someone with him on my arm? That's *hot*!"

Sydney is echoing something that other couples who are strongly connected and comfortable with a little healthy flirtation report: that their partner's presence makes it *safer* for them to be flirtatious with other people. "I actually flirt *more* when I'm in a relationship because I feel safe," says Tenisha. Rather than flirting in an attempt to make up for a *lack* of connection with their partner, they're able to flirt precisely because they're *fully* connected with them.

Seeing each other through new eyes is one of the best ways for people who have been together a long time to instantly tap back into their attraction for one another. Watching each other flirt is one way to do this. In addition, couples say that when they allow themselves to be flirtatious outside their twosome, they end up flirting more with each other as well. "It keeps me in touch with that fun-loving, provocative part of me," explains Terry, "and makes it easier to be that way with my husband too."

Being able to flirt with others in healthy and respectful ways has contributed so much to our own relationship—and led to some very entertaining encounters.

I (Joe) am a competitive swimmer, and we often run into a former lover of Mali's at the competitions we attend. Jeremy is a tall, sculpted Adonis type who is happily married to a delightful woman. We cheer each other on and stretch out on towels between races, talking about our lives and families. I actually like it when we show up at a meet and Jeremy's there too. Our friendly rivalry—and Mali and Jeremy's occasionally flirtatious friendship—definitely motivates me to swim faster when he's in the lane next to me!

On one particular sunny day, as Mali and I were hanging out on the grass between events, Jeremy snuck up on Mali from behind and squeezed her tightly at the waist. "I love these hips!" he growled. She shrieked, and we all burst out laughing. If I had chosen to be bothered by his antics, to make up some story about what they meant—like, "She'd rather be with Jeremy right now"—it wouldn't have been nearly as fun, then or now. "Hey, *Jeremy* likes these hips!" Mali will tease me every once in a while. I can tell you that when someone appreciates something about your partner that you haven't been fully appreciating, it makes you see that something in a whole new light! You instantly overcome the phenomenon that psychologists call *habituation*, which is the tendency we all have to stop noticing things because we see them so often.

I also very much enjoy it when Mali has a little crush on someone, like the good-looking spin-class instructor at our gym. It's really cute to see her acting like a nervous, tongue-tied teenager. If we take class together, I'll catch her eye and smile. It's fun to have this little secret between us! Or there's the cashier who's two decades younger than Mali and obviously has a thing for her. Going through his checkout line gives her a glow. This little interaction is energizing for her—which means it's energizing for *us*.

Before we move on, we'd like to reemphasize two very important points.

First, you and your partner should be in full agreement about this topic before experimenting, having had lots of conversations about how you each feel and what's comfortable for each of you. If this isn't something you're doing together, in complete alignment, don't do it!

Second, the intention here is never to deceive someone into thinking you're available when you're not. If you smile at a friendly face in line and have a fun little conversation, how can you be absolutely sure they aren't hoping you might be available? You can't. But if they were actually to ask you out, you can be very gracious and say thank you, but you're in a happy relationship already. This is really no different from engaging in healthy, no-agenda flirtation when you're single. There are plenty of people who are naturally flirtatious and it doesn't mean they want to go home with everyone they interact with!

Bringing the Energy of Attraction Home

We'd like to share a few more stories about how couples, including us, have used the energy of attraction to their relationship's benefit.

By the time we were writing about the topic of jealousy for *The Soulmate Experience*, I (Mali) had been practicing these ideas for so long that the process we describe earlier in this chapter (in the section "Taking Charge of Jealousy") was second nature to me. Because it was so automatic, I was finding it difficult to explain the approach in detail. I didn't realize that what I needed was a refresher course. Well, I certainly got one.

We were staying at a retreat center where we could focus on our writing in a beautiful location, with delicious food, and yoga every afternoon between our daytime and evening writing sessions. This is the kind of place where you can feel a certain level of receptivity from almost everyone you meet.

The late afternoon light was streaming through the spiraling timbers and skylight of the circular yoga structure known as The Temple. We started class sitting in a circle, eyes closed, singing a simple meditative chant to settle us into our bodies. I felt myself relaxing and breathing more deeply, a welcome letting go after a long day huddled together over our manuscript.

The chanting finished with a long, harmonious *OM*. We slowly opened our eyes.

As the circle of about ten of us stood to begin class, I noticed that Joe happened to be positioned directly across from a stunning young woman. Her blonde waves and the sunlight streaming in through the rafters caressed her tanned skin, which was set off by her saffron-colored halter top and sarong. She looked like she'd stepped right out of a "Most Naturally Beautiful Women in the World" photo essay.

Their eyes met, and as I'd always reassured him was my preference in such a situation, Joe didn't look away. Several times over the next hour, I saw them momentarily hold each other's gaze and smile. The wave of heat I was feeling in my body was definitely *not* kundalini energy rising up through my chakras. This was full-blown jealousy, with an intensity I hadn't felt in many years.

Even in my jealous fog, I realized the perfection of the situation I found myself in. I now had all the motivation I needed to review the process we'd developed for working with the insecurities and fears that can provoke jealousy in a situation like this one.

First, rather than trying to stuff down the torrent of emotions I was feeling—a jumble of panic, embarrassment, and dread—I let myself experience them. This required consciously letting go of the idea that I should be beyond jealousy by now and accepting the redness I could feel in my face. This isn't an easy thing to do, even for someone who's practiced at it. Second, I reminded myself that it wasn't Joe's *behavior* causing my distress, but what I was *telling* myself about his behavior. And third, I identified my specific "I'm not enough" beliefs playing out here: "I'm not young enough" and "I'm not beautiful enough." Even though these weren't clearly formed thoughts, I could sense them in the background, doing their best to make me feel insecure and undesirable. As one pose moved into the next, I began to silently—and emphatically!—chant more positive thoughts to myself: "Joe appreciating someone else's beauty doesn't mean I'm not enough. I'm beautiful just the way I am. And Joe loves me like crazy!"

Sweet relief. It was working! My tumultuous insides were settling down. I could now put my attention on the cool touch of the red clay floor beneath my feet, which helped me to feel more grounded. I looked around the room, appreciating the one-of-a-kind beauty of the structure we were practicing in.

Class was winding down. We stood in the circle, eyes closed, hands in front of our hearts. Namaste. *OM*.

It was over. And I was exhausted!

Though the yoga class hadn't been the restorative experience I'd been anticipating, I was happy—and relieved!—that the techniques worked. I'd been able to quiet the jealousy-producing thoughts, and I now had the personal experience I needed to write about this process in a more helpful way. I was also gratified that Joe hadn't felt compelled to avoid the radiant vision across the room, which would have been awkward and near-impossible. I was so looking forward to having dinner and talking over the experience with him.

As I was tucking my mat and yoga props back into the bins, I realized that Joe and the golden goddess weren't putting their things away with the rest of us. Instead, they had walked from their places at opposite edges of the circle until they met at the center of the room. They now stood face to face, directly beneath the skylight, talking quietly.

The jealousy roared back up even more intensely than before. While the younger version of me might have rushed forward at this point to protect her interests, my first instinct was quite the opposite, as I was determined not to let jealousy get the best of me. I reminded myself to not let jealousy control my behavior and, if at all possible, to give myself time to look at where my reaction was coming from before responding.

I ducked outside to stand in the last patches of sunlight and breathe in the soothing smells of the late California summer. I listened intently to what my crazy-making mind was trying to get me to believe. Here's what I heard: "He wishes he were single so he could explore something with her." "They're interested in each other. I should leave and let them have some space." Those thoughts were definitely the source of the heat I was feeling. I countered them with, "Joe loves me, he loves being here with me. Having attractions to others is natural. And he's coming back to the cabin with *me* tonight!" I had to repeat these firmly to myself for several minutes to unwind the knot in my stomach.

When I stepped back inside the Temple, Joe smiled and waved me over. Lovingly he put his arms around me as he introduced me to Maria, who was Swedish (of course she was), twenty-five, and traveling the world for a year on her own.

Joe said he'd told Maria about the book we were working on. He'd also explained to her that even though we love each other like crazy, and in fact can't imagine a relationship more connected and more fun than ours, we both understand that it's natural for us to be attracted to others from time to time. That's why he knew it was okay that he and Maria had taken a few minutes to talk and just experience being in each other's presence.

In her sweet Scandinavian accent, Maria told me how much she admired that I could allow the space for them to simply feel the attraction that was there between them, to look each other in the eyes and appreciate one another as beautiful souls.

I said I was grateful to them both for creating this perfect storm to compel me to remember and use the tools for working with jealousy.

Joe was taken by surprise at that. Since he'd never seen me really jealous before, it hadn't even occurred to him that I might be feeling that way!

I stood in the center of the Temple with these two "beautiful souls"—her words described them perfectly. I felt exhilarated that we were able to have such an experience and conversation.

Then a thought occurred to me. I turned to Maria.

"When you saw Joe across the circle, what did you see?"

She looked back to Joe for a few moments, then very thoughtfully answered my question. "Your boyfriend is a handsome man, but what really caught my attention was his energy. It is so warm and inviting. And he has those beautiful blue eyes, but it is the kindness in them that drew me in."

She and I both turned to him now, and all that she said was true. By sharing her perspective, Maria had given me a rare gift. As I stood looking at Joe through her eyes, I found myself re-experiencing my initial and very intense attraction to him.

Now, I know that the way this played out is a little unusual! If Joe and I hadn't had the understanding that attractions to others are natural and will come up in the course of our relationship—and without all the conversations we've had around that, and without the tools for defusing jealousy—I would probably have grabbed Joe and bolted for the exit the moment class ended, feeling hurt, angry, and embarrassed. It's also important here to highlight the fact that when Joe began speaking with Maria, he let her know right away that I was his partner. He wanted to make sure she wouldn't think he was available when he wasn't.

Joe has a little more to add to this story.

When I (Joe) saw Maria standing across the circle from me, I felt an instant connection with her. I also felt grateful that, because Mali is who she is, I wouldn't have to pretend this beautiful woman and I hadn't noticed each other or crank my neck around at odd angles all through class to avoid meeting her gaze. In my experience, mutual attractions like this don't show up all that often, so it's validating just to know they can still happen. That Mali and I can allow each other to experience them when they do arise also confirms just how cool *our* relationship is!

To let this attraction just play out, to be able to express, receive, and enjoy it, was not only an amazing experience. It also felt complete. Over the rest of the weekend, I wasn't thinking about Maria. I wasn't wondering where she was or if I'd see her again. The few times I spotted her, there was no longing, no pull to try to make something happen with her, as there might have been if I'd had to keep myself from looking in her direction and if we hadn't been able to acknowledge the attraction we'd felt between us. I would have left that class with a pent-up feeling of something unfinished.

This was a profound confirmation for me that allowing a friendly expression of mutual attraction once in a while minimizes any desire to pursue something on my own. Why would I do that and mess up the great thing we've got? If we have to hide any attractions we might experience, it creates an energetic "charge" that's completely separate from our partner. With an ongoing dialogue and clear intentions, we can consciously channel any energy of attraction that's generated *outside* our relationship right back *into* our relationship.

When Mali sends me off to the grocery store with, "Smile at someone today!" shopping is more fun, and we're super connected during that time. It's a way of activating the energy of attraction and harnessing its erotic power. She *wants* me to come home recharged. She *wants* to hear that I had a fun interaction with someone in line. Even when there's very little to tell, she likes me to stretch out the story, to tease her with it. Sometimes she seems disappointed if I *don't* have anything to tell her!

We're not the only couple who capitalizes on the energy of attraction to their relationship's advantage.

Robert talks about a personal trainer at the gym where he works out. "We've had this little flirtation going for several years. It's fun and playful, and I know we both look forward to it. She's a single mom, busy with school and work, and says it reminds her she's still an attractive woman. And she's fascinated by the fact that I tell Vanessa everything. She says she'd love to have a relationship like that one day." When Robert shares these experiences with Vanessa, the energy around his attraction shifts to *her*. Vanessa says. "We can actually feel that 'attraction energy' *through* each other."

Corrine started up a correspondence with a college boyfriend she had reconnected with through social media. Corrine's husband Edward could tell she was excited because she was putting considerable thought into her messages to the guy, reminiscing about all the adventures they'd had together. "I could have dwelled on the idea that this was bad because *I* wasn't getting this kind of attention from her," Edward says. "But it didn't take anything away from me. Just the opposite. I *liked* seeing that flirty, vivacious side of her come out." Edward says they had more flirtatious interactions themselves—and more sex—during that time than they'd had in years, and that he wouldn't be opposed to Corrine reconnecting with another old flame in the future!

Megan, a teacher and mother of a toddler, was away at a weekend conference and found herself seated next to a very handsome man at dinner. "I enjoyed the wine and the attention," she says, "and that feeling like I was single again." When Megan returned to her room that evening, she called her husband and told him all about her night. "Zack and I had phone sex—the first time ever for both of us!" she laughs. When dinnertime came around the next evening, Megan coyly seated herself near the man again. She had a great time, excusing herself before dessert so she'd have time for an extended phone date with Zack. Having the opportunity to enjoy this man's attentions added a fun new dimension to her sex life with her husband. Zack says, "We're grateful to him, even if she never sees him again!"

These couples all understand that our erotic batteries can get charged up by more than just our partner and that we don't have to discharge that energy with anyone *other* than our partner. By intentionally bringing any energy of attraction that gets activated back home to our relationship, our relationship continues to be where the excitement is and where we both want to stay and play.

7

PLAYING IN THE GARDEN OF EDEN: MORE IDEAS FOR INTIMATE ADVENTURES

We've covered a diverse range of approaches that we believe can help keep a long-term relationship sexually satisfying. We've explored ways to turn insecurities, inhibitions, and performance issues into opportunities for intimacy. We've delved into how couples might allow their individual interests and past experiences to fuel their sexual connection. And we've demystified how "just enough jealousy" can be channeled into passion and desire. But what does science have to say about it?

Several studies have confirmed that couples who say their sex life has remained passionate over time have certain attitudes and behaviors in common.[1] Here's the shortlist of things that couples who have more fulfilling sex lives do—or do more frequently—than couples who are less satisfied with their sex lives:

- Communicate openly about sex, such as their desires or their likes and dislikes
- Engage in sexy talk, texts, or emails
- Have a positive attitude toward sexuality

- Set the mood for a romantic or sexual encounter, such as by lowering the lights and putting on music
- Make intimacy and romance a priority, whether through kissing, cuddling, touching, laughing together during sex, or saying "I love you"
- Talk about and act out fantasies
- Take time for more foreplay, longer sexual encounters, and romantic getaways
- Experiment with new locations, positions, and activities
- Mix it up by incorporating such things as massage, lingerie, light bondage, anal play, and sex toys
- Enjoy oral sex, both giving and receiving

The authors of one of the largest studies of this kind concluded that, "If properly nurtured, passion can last for decades."[2]

More than anything, this list highlights the idea that one of the best ways to nurture passion is simply by having an open, adventurous mindset toward sex. It's in this spirit that we'd like to suggest you start thinking not of being in a long-term *relationship*, but of being on a long-term *adventure*.

PANDORA AND EVE WERE FRAMED

In Greek mythology, Pandora opened a container that was supposedly filled with all the world's evils. In the Old Testament, Eve was tempted by the serpent into eating the forbidden fruit from the tree of knowledge of good and evil in the Garden of Eden. These two women were to be eternally blamed for allowing curiosity to get the better of them and bringing trouble into the world.

The idea that women are the source of all the world's evils is obviously preposterous. Yet a common thread in these stories, especially as it relates to sexuality, does have validity: that women are inherently curious. Although people of all genders have the capacity to be curious and open to new experiences, studies show that women are typically more erotically adventurous than men and are naturally turned on by a greater variety of things than men are.[3] When it comes to keeping a relationship sexually inspired, curiosity isn't a liability. It's an asset!

It's time to reinterpret these myths and give curiosity and an adventurous spirit the respect they deserve. Let's look at it this way: Eve and Pandora weren't bringing trouble into the world, they were bringing *possibilities*.

Bring your sense of adventure and a willingness to play to the collection of ideas in this chapter for keeping sex fresh and fun. You and your lover will very likely have different levels of interest in or comfort with many of these suggestions, so remember that you don't have to say yes to everything. But do say yes to *something*! And reassure each other that anytime you step too far out of your comfort zones, you can choose to step right back in.

Get Your Hearts Thumping

Exciting new experiences cause the body to produce adrenaline, the same hormone that's activated when we felt those first rushes of sexual attraction to each other. So go beyond "dinner and a movie" by experimenting with activities that are new to you both. With ten minutes of research—try "exciting date ideas" or listings of local events—you'll find plenty of opportunities for a little adventure.

Take a class together, like salsa dancing, hula hooping, or couple's massage. Join a drum circle, go out for karaoke, eat at a "dine in the dark" restaurant, brave a zip line, or shoot a game at the local pool hall. Physical activities, particularly unfamiliar ones, are especially bonding, as they will call on you to support one another. Try partner yoga, a hip-hop class, or indoor skydiving, or take lessons at a rock-climbing gym. And those times you do opt for dinner and a movie, try choosing the restaurant for its sensual food and atmosphere and the film for its breathtaking cinematography or epic music.

Spice Up Date Night

Setting aside time for a regular date night is common advice for couples wanting to keep their overall relationship vibrant. If we want to maintain vibrancy in our sex life, we need more than just date nights. We need *sexy* date nights!

Susan sometimes gives her husband the task of keeping her nipples hard when they're out for dinner. He might kiss her shoulder, blow in her ear, or secretly squeeze one of her breasts while giving her a hug. "It drives me absolutely crazy!" she says.

Consider going out with each of you taking on a new identity. This is your chance to be that famous novelist, international spy, or renowned winemaker. We've laughed for years about the day Mali told some guy we were chatting with in a beer garden that she used to be a famous stripper down in Florida and that twenty dollars of polyester put her through college.

Check event listings for sensual art exhibits or performances. If this suggestion has one of you feeling insecure, as you'll be inclined to compare yourself to the artwork or performers and feel insufficient, your partner can remind you, "We're here for *us*, to enjoy this show *together*."

Or stay at home and catch a sophisticated, sexually explicit television series. Search "sexiest TV shows" or "best documentaries about sex" for ideas. You might also look for empowering documentaries that explore an issue that affects one of you personally, such as erectile dysfunction, premature ejaculation, sexual shyness, or concerns about penis, vulva, or breast size or shape. There are also educational sites that feature instructional videos on everything from sexual communication to self-pleasuring to oral sex techniques.

Finally, wholeheartedly indulge yourselves in sensual pleasures. Take a walk by the light of the moon. Feed each other with your fingers. Bathe or swim naked together. Take a blindfolded shower or hot tub. Or hold a wet t-shirt contest for one—or for you both!

Beautify Your Boudoir

Another standard piece of advice for couples is to find unusual places to have sex. But even if you do manage this on occasion, you'll probably still be spending most of your sexy time in the bedroom. So give a little attention to setting the scene.

Create an ambiance for intimacy: make the bed, dust, and sweep or vacuum. Having places to quickly tuck away the clutter and electronics can help you keep surfaces clear. And for sex's sake, don't forget to give the bathroom a quick sprucing up!

Invest in some decent sheets, towels, and speakers, along with a cozy comforter or soft throw blanket. Decorate with things you love, perhaps picking out sensual photographs or art together. For a little natural beauty, consider bringing in a plant or flowers. Add romance with soft lighting, candles, and an essential oil diffuser—some people get aroused by vanilla, sandalwood, musk, or citrus scents. For extra visual stimulation and more opportunities for intimate eye contact, hang a mirror or have one available you can strategically place when the moments arise. And finally, for maximum comfort and creativity, make sure to have a few firm pillows on hand.

Designate a Sex Box and Fill It with Toys

Stash away some sexy playtime accoutrements in a special drawer or—in honor of Pandora!—a secret sex box.

Massagers and body oils are wonderful for getting in the mood. There's an endless variety of massagers for every area of the body—like those shaped specifically for the neck or for kneading out knots in the back. Using them on each other can help you relax, let go of pain, and be more present.

So many everyday objects can be used for sensual play, like spatulas, bandanas, neckties, textured bath gloves, feathers, and clothespins. Walk around your house in search of such "pervertibles" together. You'll be opening drawers and cupboards with new eyes! And don't toss that flirtatious dress or muscle shirt just because you think you've outgrown it. If you still feel sexy in it—or your lover gets turned on seeing you in it!—tuck it into the sex box too.

On date night, visit an adult toy store with a positive vibe and explore the ever-expanding world of sex toys, from restraints to crystal wands, slings to sex pillows, strap-ons to cock rings. Or peruse some online pleasure toyshops. There are lots of wonderful ones to choose from, many with a special focus on women's comfort and pleasure. You might choose masturbation toys for each of you, to use together and on each other. Also check out the sex toys couples can use for simultaneous stimulation. And be sure to investigate all the sexy extras, like clip-on jewelry for nipples, navels, and other fun places.

Some people oppose masturbation toys for various reasons, so let's dispel some of those concerns. Despite what some women might fear, a masturbation sleeve for a male partner doesn't mean he's looking to replace her. If, however, he seems to consistently prefer masturbating to making love, there are probably larger issues in the relationship that could use addressing.

If you worry that you'll become dependent on a vibrator, just be sure to continue exploring your own arousal and pleasure in many different ways. An orgasm from an unexpected source could be just around the corner! For some vulva owners, vibrators can stimulate internal clitoral tissues in ways that a hand, mouth, or penis simply can't. Some women like that type of stimulation to help them climax, while others just enjoy the additional sensations. And vibrators can be put to imaginative use to create tingles and shivers all over the body.

Finally, if you've been conditioned to believe that you should be able to provide your partner with enough pleasure that they don't "need" a vibrator, understand that your partner enjoying a vibrator doesn't make you less of a lover. In fact, being open to whatever brings your partner pleasure makes you *more* of a lover. You could even eroticize this insecurity by searching together for toys, and ways to play with them, that *really* get each of you off!

Return to the Scene of the Pleasure

We're often more experimental when we're newly dating. Reminisce about any sexy adventures you've already had together and consider re-creating those scenes when you have the opportunity.

Alex and Taylor used to have sex in the backseat of their car in their own driveway out of necessity. Their house was small and their children were light sleepers. They've done it a few times since just to reconnect with the risky feeling that excited them back then.

When Joe and I (Mali) were first dating, he often traveled locally for business. I'd sometimes meet him at his hotel room in the evening, where he'd be waiting in a suit and tie. He looked so masculine and sexy, I'd hardly make it through the door before jumping on him. He rarely wears suits now, but I occasionally coax him into dressing up in one at home. He's always willing, as he knows it won't stay on for long!

Make Love to Music

Music can be a great accompaniment to making out or making love, so have fun getting down to all different styles: reggae, classical, blues, Afrobeat, country, rock, soul, EDM. Leave any "this ain't my genre" objections at the door and see if there's something you *can* appreciate about what you're hearing. If you find lyrics distracting, try instrumental tracks or selections in a language you don't know.

You might discover that the romantic rhythms and passionate melodies of a Spanish guitar create the perfect ambiance for an evening's lovemaking. Or that the soulful vibrations of the cello encourage your lover to take their sweet time as you lie back and enjoy their attention. A particularly hypnotic hip-hop jam might inspire some serious tongue exploration, while the repetitive beat of a techno or trance track can propel you into a rhythmic groove.

Give each other opportunities to play your own favorites for giving or receiving head. And if you're feeling brave, discover some new artists by swapping sex playlists with your friends!

Treat Each Other to a Sensual Massage

Massage is a wonderful way to set the mood and reconnect. The focus in the following is on massaging a woman, but a similar approach would work for anyone.

Warm up the room, put on some soft music, and light a candle or two. Have her undress and lie facedown, draped with a sheet. Offer to place a pillow under her hips or feet. Tell her, "For the next hour, your only requirement is to relax and enjoy. If something doesn't feel right, or feels especially good, or if you have any sore or tender spots, I'd love to know."

Start by gently running your hands over her entire body to awaken her senses. Then pull the sheet aside, uncovering one area at a time to receive your attention. Experiment with a soft touch as well as with longer, firmer strokes, applying oil if she'd like. When you find something she particularly enjoys, stay there and *indulge her*!

If any part of her body is tense or aching, kiss and caress that area. Her butt and upper thighs are erogenous regions that many massages don't include, so spend some time rhythmically squeezing and releasing the muscles in her lower back, ass cheeks, and upper thighs. Before inviting her to turn over, ask if there is any place she'd like you to focus a little more attention.

Lift the sheet for her as she rolls onto her back. Begin this part of the massage by lightly tracing your fingers from her face down to her toes and back again a few times. Spend time on her face, caressing her cheeks and jaw line, kissing her forehead and eyes, massaging her scalp, gently tugging her ears. Massaging her belly in a circular motion can be intimate and relaxing.

Slowly turn your attention to other erogenous zones like her neck, ears, hips, and inner thighs. Many people find it exquisite to have their entire breasts held and massaged, especially if they've been restrained in a bra all week long. The undersides of her breasts may rarely get touched. When you explore her nipples, start gently and let her responses guide you as you love them into attention. Some women never like their nipples touched directly, in which case you might just kiss around the areolas or blow warm air over them.

When you move your loving touch to her genital area, your goal is not necessarily to bring her to orgasm, but to help her experience as much sensuality and pleasure as possible. Remind her that she's welcome to guide you (or stop you!) at any time. Some women, for example, don't like direct stimulation of the clitoris.

Build sensation and anticipation by slowly moving toward her most sensitive areas. Many women find the feeling of cupping—holding the entire genital area, from perineum to pubic bone, with one or both hands—both nurturing and arousing. Try this gently at first and then with more pressure.

Look for signs that she's getting turned on as you play with stroking, teasing, and caressing her: a moan, a sigh, a flush, the swelling of her breasts or vulva. When you're fully tuned in, you will more easily discover what kinds of attention will bring her the most pleasure.

If the person you're massaging is a man, this could be a rare opportunity for him to just lie back and receive. You might acknowledge from the start that he may or may not get an erection at various points during the massage, and either is just fine. When you do move to his genitals, spend as much time on the surrounding areas as on the penis itself. Just having his testicles held and gently manipulated can feel delicious, as can massaging the parts of the penis that are buried beneath the surface. Let him know there's no expectation that he gets hard. His only job is to enjoy the sensations, whether he gets an erection or not!

A sweet finishing touch is to simply hold your lover, for as long as they would like to be held.

Get Naked Together

If either of you isn't fully at ease naked, this is a great opportunity to support each other's growth and healing. Start with an intimate conversation: *What did you each learn about nudity growing up? How comfortable are you being naked when you're alone, when it's just the two of you? How about when you're with other people? What might help you become more comfortable?* What you're discovering is where your edges are and where you might stretch a little. For some people, just sleeping naked would be a big stretch.

You might walk together around your bedroom or home without clothes on, or even turn the lights down and dance. Water, especially warm water, can be very soothing. If you have access to a large bathtub or hot tub, you can float your lover in your arms. Make sure their nose remains above the surface and that their ears stay dry if water bothers them. Allow your lover to completely relax while every inch of their body is being supported by either you or the water.

When you're traveling, look for opportunities to be naked, such as the communal bathhouses and spas in Japan, Korea, or Europe or the clothing-optional hot springs across the United States. You can always start with a swimsuit and remove it when you're feeling more comfortable. Being nude around other people in nonsexual environments can be surprisingly liberating. If you're feeling nervous, remember to focus on the sensations you're experiencing and on the feeling of freedom when you're unrestricted by clothing, rather than on any thoughts about how your body might look.

Keep the Sexy Surprises Coming

Take your lover on a treasure hunt for the shirt, dress, or sleepwear that looks the hottest on them. For you reluctant shoppers out there, don't think of this as shopping. Think of it as foreplay! If you don't find anything this time, that's just fine, as it gives you a reason to play the role of their dedicated personal shopper again.

Visit a lingerie or sensuality store and check out the sexy accessories: stockings, stick-on tattoos, body paint, and jewelry. There's a whole world of nonpiercing jewelry for adorning all areas of the body, like navels, nipples, lips, and vulvas. Or get your hands on a kit for creating a silicone replica of you or your partner's (formerly) private parts—which you can also turn into a vibrating version!

For a special occasion, consider a sensual experience like a foot reflexology session or a massage for two. Rashona took her lover Zain to Las Vegas to have her painted and photographed by a professional body painter.

A sexy surprise doesn't have to be pricey. Martin's most cherished gift from his girlfriend Leila didn't cost her a cent. She had marked a map with an X in all the locations they've had a good time together, and with a heart sticker where they've had a *really* good time together. "Looking at the map keeps us inspired to keep adding to it," Leila says. "Like our road trips. We keep an eye out for places to pull off the road for a little fooling around. We've learned that our GPS can tell us where we are, but it can't tell us how much fun we're having!"

Keep the Sexy Dialogue Going

Sexy texts and conversations can keep your juices flowing. Here are a few seductive conversation starters: "I'm thinking about that time we . . ." "When you're naked, I love checking out your . . ." "I've been imagining us . . ." "Do you have any idea how much I love your . . . ?"

Or put a sexy overtone on an everyday comment. Just speak in a playful way while giving your partner a flirtatious glance: "Ooo, this orange is really juicy!"

Some people don't like any talking at all after the kissing begins, but we'd like to persuade you to try it, as it can amplify your erotic connection. If you feel silly or inauthentic, just put into words whatever hot thoughts you're thinking: "It turns me on to see you in those tight jeans!" "When I get you naked, I'm going to . . ." "I want you to use me!" "I know exactly how you like this." Or describe what you're experiencing: "Squeezing your ass is really getting me hot!" "Watching you take your shirt off makes me want you." "When you run your hands over my chest like that, it makes my nipples hard." "The smell of your sweaty skin is making me so wet."

If you can't imagine saying anything like this aloud, how about whispering it?

You might try playing with a little verbal dominance. Be directive: "Undress, slowly, while I watch from over here." "I want you to lie back, spread your legs, and wait for me." "Don't try to rush me. I'm going to take my sweet time here!" "Turn around, get in position, and I'm going to do that thing you love—when I'm good and ready!" "I want to watch you come for me!" Or you can be a little submissive or naughty: "My body is all yours tonight. Use me for your pleasure!" "Tell me what you want me to do." "I've been bad today. . . ."

Yes, you can feel awkward or self-conscious saying—and hearing—these kinds of things if you're not used to it. But seriously, what's the worst that could happen if you experience a little awkwardness? This is a place to take a little risk, to stretch your comfort zones, and that's a good thing—we want those opportunities. Besides, your inhibitions will tend to lessen as you get more turned on.

Even if the two of you just end up laughing together, that's okay too. Laughter is one of the best aphrodisiacs around, and it will help you stop worrying about how silly you sound!

You might also have a conversation in which you each answer these questions: *What could your lover say that would turn you on?* (This doesn't have to be standard porn dirty talk. It could be that you want to hear how much you are loved or desired.) *How would hearing those words make you feel? Are there particular times you'd like to hear that? And what kinds of things do you find it exciting or sexy to say—and how does saying those words make you feel?*

Oh, and one more idea. Have fun giving each other a secret sex name. And no, even though their origin stories are pretty hilarious, we're not going to tell you ours!

Play with PDAs

Public displays of affection, like holding hands, hugging, or kissing when others are nearby, come quite naturally to some people, depending on the situation. Other people, often because of where or how they were raised, can feel uncomfortable with PDAs no matter the circumstances. If you've always been uneasy with expressions of affection in public, and especially if your partner *is* comfortable with them, it might be an erotic edge for you to play at. Before you start shaking your head, we want to be clear that we're not advocating for SDAs, or sexual displays of affection.

When you're waiting in line for a movie or hanging out at the corner pub, stand with your arms around one another, massage each other's neck or shoulders, or experiment with a simple kiss. While it's true that someone might roll their eyes at you for being "that couple," we can attest that many people can be inspired by seeing couples who are playfully affectionate.

Try On Other People's Turn-Ons

In chapter 3, we suggested that the sexual interests and fantasies of other people are an endless source of new ideas to experiment with. Almost anything someone might be into—whether it's high heels, jockstraps, silk, leather, latex, or maple syrup—can give you ideas. It doesn't have to be *your* fantasy for the two of you to have some fun with it.

One of my (Mali's) favorites that we've explored so far is puppy play, an interest that involves role-playing being a dog. When Joe drops down on his hands and knees and starts nipping and tugging at me like I'm his best puppy friend, or chewing on my neck like I'm his toy, his silly antics and puppy growls send shivers and giggles through my body. Being open to this particular turn-on means that every now and then, I get some sweet puppy love!

Be Each Other's Object of Desire

In *What Do Women Want? Adventures in the Science of Female Desire*, author Daniel Bergner makes the case that a central component of women's desire is, in essence, to be desired. In *Not Always in the Mood: The New Science of Men, Sex, and Relationships*, sexuality researcher Sarah Hunter Murray asserts that feeling desired is a primary factor affecting men's interest in having sex with a long-term partner.

Pretty much everyone, it seems, wants to feel desired, even people who are usually the ones to initiate sexual activity. So create some opportunities for each of you to be the other's object of desire.

If the thought of being on display makes you squirm but your partner is supportive, this is a chance to enjoy some risqué play while developing more self-confidence. The basic idea is for one of you to just relax back and admire your lover as they seductively move or even dance for you.

Watch some videos on tips for giving a striptease or lap dance. You might even take a burlesque, stripping, or pole-dancing class, which are terrific exercise as well. Then lower the lights, play some music that inspires you, and put that sexy apparel you've collected to use. If it helps, close your eyes at first to focus on feeling the rhythms and melodies in your body. Allow yourself to begin to move with them, without worrying about how you look. You also may want to try incorporating some sensual interaction into your performance, like pleasuring yourself, pleasuring your audience, or offering them the opportunity to pleasure you. Rather than focusing on being "good" at this, just have fun with it!

If you're the lucky audience, reassure your lover that you don't expect them to be a professional dancer and that you'll love anything they do. Remind them that this is a safe place for them to let go of self-consciousness, a place to feel sexy and have a little fun. We often view a partner's body with more acceptance and appreciation than they do themselves. So you might describe what you're seeing that turns you on as your lover takes in what you're saying as your truth (no arguing allowed!).

I (Mali) enjoy dressing up and performing for Joe. It indulges my femininity, my seductive side, and my love of sexy clothing and music. To stretch the tease out, I'll sometimes put on several pairs of panties, thigh-high stockings, leggings, a belly chain, a bustier over a lacy bra, a couple of sexy belts, a silky scarf, and a blouse, skirt, and jacket to top it all off. Every time I begin, it takes me a while to shake off my self-consciousness. Joe helps by reminding me that whatever I do will be appreciated. And yes, he's also willing to treat me to this voyeuristic fun too, even though this is far more of an edge for him. Dancing for each other makes us both feel more confident, and it's very sexy to be so desired by the object of *your* desire!

Here's one more way to help your lover experience themselves as an object of lust and desire: touch them sensuously while they relax in front of a mirror and take in their own image as an erotic art form.

Put Sex on the Calendar

If your lives revolve around schedules, homework, and your children's play dates, leave the kids with the neighbors and have a play date yourselves once in a while—a sex play date! If you're worried that planning for sex will strip away the fun, think back to when you were first together and you'll remember that anticipation was a big *part* of the fun. As sexologists Jessica O'Reilly and Marla Renee Stewart write in *The Ultimate Guide to Seduction and Foreplay*, "Anticipation is not the precursor to pleasure; *anticipation is pleasure*." Raymond, who's been dating Mandy for several years, agrees. "It's all about the buildup," he says. "I love thinking about an upcoming date, texting each other in the days before—I'm thinking about you in that red skirt, I'd love to do this to you." Raymond says it doesn't even matter if they actually do what they've been scheming about when they finally get together. "It's the sexual tension we're creating that's so exciting!" he explains.

When you have the time, squeeze in an entire sex weekend. Leave behind your roles as spouses, parents, and wage earners and come back together as lovers. A sex vacation isn't about going somewhere with a sightseeing itinerary, but with your imagination, a few intimate accessories, and an intention to love each other up. This can include enjoying some sensual food, a romantic picnic, a titillating movie, or a couple's massage.

If you just can't get away but your kids are old enough to occupy themselves for a while, take some private time for yourselves in your bedroom. It's positive role-modeling for them to see their parents treat their own relationship as a priority.

Take a Hands-On Approach

Fingers and hands are amazing, and so versatile. Knowing this, either of you might enjoy being treated to a session of hand sex, or sexual stimulation using just the hands. Well, hands and maybe some erotic massage oil, which you can easily make yourself (maybe as a gift for your lover!).

Get into comfortable positions. Pillows can be helpful. You might ask if there's any particular music your lover would like to hear. To build anticipation, start your attentions through their clothing. Apply some pressure until they feel the warmth of your hands through the fabric. Let them know they're welcome to guide you at any time. For example, they might say, "How about trying this?" "That's a little too sensitive." "Before we get really into that—which feels awesome—could we circle back to what you were doing just before?" "Oh yes, keep doing that—just like that!"

Get creative—this isn't a hand *job*, it's a hand *exploration*! Experiment with different grips and strokes, try twisting and spiraling motions, and vary the speed and pressure. The entire region is an erogenous zone, so involve nearby areas in the fun: the inner thighs, the perineum, the testicles, the anal area. If there's music playing, try tapping, squeezing, or stroking in sync with the rhythms. When you find something your partner particularly enjoys, stay there for a while. Give them time to settle into how good it's feeling.

If your lover has a vagina and welcomes internal stimulation, start slowly and keep up the communication. Explore the sensitivities of the various areas, trying one, two, or more fingers and experimenting with swirling, rocking, and rotating motions. Notice how different the muscles and tissues are around the opening from how they are further in. There are various pressure and pleasure points to discover, including, perhaps, a zone of soft tissue and increased sensitivity along the vagina's front wall, typically referred to as the G-spot. While only about one-quarter of the entire clitoral structure is visible outside the body (the part commonly called "the clitoris"), a good part of the internal portion wraps up and around the vagina. So it makes sense that pressure through the vaginal wall could stimulate the clitoris from the inside. As sex therapist Ian Kerner writes in *She Comes First: The Thinking Man's Guide to Pleasuring a Woman*, "A G-spot orgasm, like all female orgasms, is a clitoral orgasm; it's part of the same pleasure network." Pressure in this area could also involve stimulation of the spongy erectile tissue that surrounds the urethra.[4] Whether exploring this area or elsewhere, have fun on this pleasure hunt!

At any time during your hand-sex session, looking into each other's eyes can be particularly sexy and connecting.

Have Some Backdoor Fun

Though still a taboo in many contexts, anal sex has made it into mainstream shows and movies over the past couple of decades. For some couples, that taboo factor is precisely what makes ass play so exciting.

Anal play isn't limited to deep penetration. There are many nerve endings around the opening and just inside, which means many opportunities for new sensations and pleasure. In addition, plenty of people find that certain kinds of pressure from the inside feels exquisite, as it stimulates their prostate gland or internal clitoral tissues (the parts of the clitoris that extend inside the body).

This is an extremely sensitive area that needs to be approached with gentleness and care. So before diving in, do some research together for tips on choosing lubricants, ensuring things are as clean as possible, and staying relaxed.

Some people find exposing themselves in this way very freeing, while others can be hesitant, in which case you can turn the lights down and offer reassurance: "I am very turned-on by the sight. It's something I associate with hot, passionate lovemaking." This could be a long exploration, over many sessions, sensual and erotic even if it never results in any kind of penetration.

Make Love to Yourselves in Front of Each Other

It can be deeply intimate to lie back and witness your lover's self-pleasure, as well as liberating to let yourself be seen in this most personal way. Some people will find they are natural exhibitionists and get very turned on pleasuring themselves for their lover, while others are natural voyeurs—watching will be just as exciting for them.

If you're the one being watched but are feeling self-conscious, do whatever it takes to relax, whether that's lowering the lights, playing some music, or enjoying a little of your favorite disinhibitor—like that champagne you saved for a special occasion. Consider asking your lover to watch from a short distance away. You might also close your eyes and try exploring your body as though it were someone else's. Run your hands over your contours, appreciate the strength in your shoulders and legs, massage your chest, enjoy the feeling of your breasts or your ass cheeks in your hands.

If you're the one watching, reassure the talent that you won't be judging, just appreciating, and that you have no expectations about how they might masturbate. If you do have expectations, drop them right now. This isn't porn, it's real life!

You might also try self-pleasuring together, intertwining your bodies in different ways and maybe even looking into each other's eyes as you orgasm. If you're not comfortable masturbating in your lover's presence the way you would if you were alone, you might be able to slowly allow yourself—with your partner's understanding and encouragement—to be more relaxed and authentically *you* over time.

Embellish Your Lip Service

We explore many creative approaches to oral sex in chapter 3. Because of its endless potential for sensual creativity and pleasure, here are a few more. Just remember that the ultimate secret to being awesome at oral is being totally into it, indulging in all the curves and textures and tastes and rhythms.

- Get things started with some "oral" around oral. Together, look up lists of "oral sex tips" or "best blowjob (or cunnilingus) techniques" and talk about which ideas intrigue or excite each of you.
- Experiment with unusual positions and locations. Ever play mermaid and try a little underwater head? Or sneak off into a closet like it's done in the movies?
- Go down on your lover without an intention to get them hard or bring them to orgasm, but just to create as many different sensations as you can. Softly massage and caress their genitals with your hands while you kiss, nibble, and suck every centimeter—listening, as always, with all of your senses to their responses and inviting their feedback.
- If your lover has a penis, give them oral while they attempt to stay soft. This can be very intimate, because it isn't what's expected (it certainly isn't what you see in porn!) and there are new and different sensations to play with.
- If your lover has a vulva, pretend that your lips are passionately making out with their lips.
- Treat your lover to a session of oral in front of a mirror so they can watch from another perspective—while connecting with your reflection.
- Have your lover create a special playlist for receiving oral sex. Incorporate the feelings and rhythms of the music into your sensual attentions.
- For a special treat, pleasure your partner while they watch a favorite sexy scene or read something they find erotic. Or, if they're into the idea, pleasure them while they're watching something *you* enjoy so that they can make an erotic connection with what excites you.

Snap Some Sexy Selfies

Most of us essentially carry around a photography studio with us wherever we go. Why not put yours to use to visually capture some of the sensuality, passion, and intimacy between you?

If the thought of being photographed makes either or both of you nervous, don't worry about posing. You'll often find that the best photos are those that portray authentic intimacy. It's okay to experiment and take a bunch of pictures and then save just one, or none. Have fun playing with cropping and filters until you get an image you really like.

Be smart, and take steps to keep your sexy selfies for your eyes only. Put your phone into airplane mode, and make sure to completely delete any images you don't want. Hide those you do want in a photo vault app or in a password-protected folder on your computer. As nothing is ever 100 percent secure, if you couldn't bear the possibility of a particular image getting into someone else's hands, don't take it. And sexy selfies don't have to be nudes. Pictures with clothing and tight cropping can be quite sexy.

Looking back at your intimate moments together, even many years later, will remind the two of you of some special memories you've made—and could very well inspire you to make new ones!

Incorporate Breath and Sound

The use of breath and sound is a core component of tantra (as it is practiced in the West) and sacred sexuality teachings. Typically taught in intimacy courses, breath and sound are tools that you can consciously use to move energy through your body and become more in tune with yourself. They will help you to quiet your busy mind and move more into your body, and to notice and pay closer attention to subtle sensations. By helping you be more present to what's happening in this moment, breathing and making sounds with awareness will make it easier to know what's feeling good and what's not.

By being more in touch with what's going on inside of you, you can also communicate that to your partner, which in itself creates intimacy. The vulnerability that's required to be emotionally expressive is erotic in its own way.

Using these tools doesn't have to be complicated or dramatic. Just making a few sighing sounds and shaking or wriggling around will relieve tension. You can actually feel it coming out of your body. Or try sighing deeply a few times while saying the sound HAAAA. Let the sound come from deep in your belly. The vibrations moving through your body can actually feel very sexy and stimulating! Put your hands over your lower belly and genital area to feel the movement of the sound. You can use this practice to bring yourself back if your mind is checking out or if you're getting overexcited and want to calm things down.

Or if you'd like to pause and reconnect, you can breathe together. Try synchronizing your breathing, or one of you can breathe in while the other breathes out. Or try belly-to-belly breathing, where you're physically connected and inhaling and exhaling in sync, your bellies expanding and contracting together. Just consciously breathing together can feel so intimate.

Making sounds together can bring more freedom into your lovemaking. Many people hold back from making sounds during sexual interactions, but being able to do so can be liberating. Give yourselves permission to experiment with sighing, moaning, and groaning, even if you think you sound weird or forced. It's okay to feel weird trying something you haven't tried before! Just breathe more deeply, keep making the sounds, and allow your whole body to get into the rhythm. There might be sounds that come from deep within you that turn you both on more than you could ever have imagined!

Explore Erotica Together

For some couples, indulging in some erotica together is fun and encourages experimentation. If watching erotica with your partner isn't something you feel ready for or interested in, or if the idea causes you to feel body anxiety or shame, consider instead seeing a softcore sexy movie or reading sexy stories to each other (try searching "erotic fiction").

If you're both okay watching some kinds of sexually explicit videos, it can be a way to share some of your interests as well as a source of new ideas. Quinn and Kerry say, "We watch all kinds of crazy stuff just for fun. It amazes us what some people are into!" Of course, if anything makes either of you feel threatened or uncomfortable, move on.

While there's an endless stream of poorly or unethically produced pornography out there, there's also more and more content that's made with integrity. Search on "consciously produced erotica," "ethical erotica," or "feminist pornography" to find content in which the actors are treated with respect and their safety and well-being are paramount. You might look for erotica that emphasizes natural bodies and authentic interactions or that's sensual, artistic, and even affectionate and loving. Such higher-quality material isn't typically free, but the modest cost is necessary to support its creation.

On the flip side, if either or both of you tend to watch a lot of porn, consider taking a break for awhile just to see what effects that might have. This could be one more way to foster a new and different experience together!

Flirt Together

In chapter 6 we explored how a little playful flirtation with others, when you both know you have nothing to fear, is a way to charge up your own erotic connection. And *watching* each other flirt can instantly intensify your attraction to and desire for one another.

If you're both intrigued by the idea, walk around an outdoor music venue or farmers' market a short distance apart, both of you feeling for that potential for connection with someone new. You might even exchange a smile or a few words with an interesting stranger.

Contemplating what another person who's attracted to your partner is seeing will have the effect of making your partner even more desirable in your eyes. "Seeing someone look at my guy with interest fires up *my* interest in him," says Riley. "I remember I'm not the only one who finds him hot!"

We can almost guarantee that being flirtatious together will make flirting with each other come more naturally and spontaneously as well.

Try Getting High

Some people advocate always being sober during sex, and mind-altering substances might not be for you, but several recent studies have confirmed that marijuana can have sensual benefits.[5] Some people use it before lovemaking to relax, relieve pain, or reduce anxiety around body-image or performance issues. Others find that marijuana highlights feelings of love and affection and helps them open up emotionally. Joanne, who's been married for three decades, says, "Enjoying a little marijuana together helps us let go of the stresses of the day and really connect." Trevor, who started using marijuana with his partner after his elderly parents moved in with them, says it's made a huge contribution to their Saturday date nights: "I'm not gonna lie. Weed saved our sex life!" At lower doses, cannabis has also been shown to promote creativity—and creativity, of course, can fire up sensual and sexual exploration.

All of these potential effects may depend on the kind and dosage, as well as your state of mind and your intention: are you using this substance to check out or to be more tuned in? You might need to experiment to know whether certain types of marijuana have an aphrodisiac effect for you or make you anxious or sleepy. If you live in or are visiting a place where cannabis is legal, ask at a dispensary which strain or blend might be best for you.

Although not yet a major focus of clinical research, there's anecdotal evidence that topical preparations of cannabis, when applied to the vulva, clitoris, or vagina, can enhance sexual arousal and orgasms. The active compounds in these products might help to relax and increase blood flow to the area, reduce pain, increase lubrication, and heighten sensitivity, all without psychological effects. Individual results will, of course, vary.

Attend an Intimacy Event or Wild Workshop

With more and more people realizing they could use some help in the intimacy arena, workshops and retreats for couples have become increasingly popular. Search for "couples intimacy retreats," "marriage workshops," or "sexuality retreats for couples" to discover what's happening in your area, somewhere you're traveling to, or somewhere you *could* travel to.

These events typically involve some combination of communication exercises and role-play, group discussions, breathing and meditation practices, movement and touching activities, and sense-opening experiences. You might do exercises to help you let go of body-image issues and self-consciousness and become more present with and attuned to each other, physically and emotionally. Many of these events offer a relaxing environment where you can spend time alone together and reconnect. You might be given sex homework to do once you're back in your private quarters.

More intimate workshops might include some degree of physical intimacy between the two of you, such as hugging, massaging, kissing, or touching activities, while you're in the group setting. Some even involve various levels of intimacy with other participants, so do your research. Ask questions, read reviews, and, if possible, talk to people who have attended to make sure the workshop feels like a good fit for the two of you.

If you go to one workshop and it's not for you, don't give up. There is such a variety of offerings available that there are bound to be some that will enrich the connection and pleasure within your relationship.

Some intimacy and tantra workshops are also available online. Lynn and Makani say this about taking a few of these together from the privacy of their own bedroom: "The results and impacts have been unexpected and very positive, helping us get more real and vulnerable and creating so much more connection."

Finally, for the even more adventurous, there are all kinds of erotic events to check out, from naked yoga classes to classes on cunnilingus or anal pleasure to female ejaculation workshops to erotic masquerade balls and sex expos. The possibilities really are endless!

Take on an Imaginary Lover—or Two!

We've talked about cultivating receptivity to each other's fantasies as well as when and how you might share them. In the right circumstances, knowing that your lover is fantasizing about someone else can have you riding that "just enough jealousy" edge, flooding your system with sexy hormones and adding to your mutual arousal and enjoyment. The same can be true for you fantasizing about your lover being with another person.

Dan and Samantha, for example, are still making love after twenty-five years and are perfectly comfortable with each other fantasizing during sex. "She can pretend I'm anyone she wants," Dan explains. "If she's having fun, I'm having fun!"

I (Joe) also sometimes fantasize that Mali is someone else while we're making love. This momentary overlay of a fantasy is like superimposing a new persona on her, but the core person, the woman I'm so in love with, is still there with me. This is very different from using a fantasy to "replace" your partner—I've been there too. In what's called a "partner replacement fantasy," you're trying to get the person you're with out of your mind by imagining them actually *being* someone else. Because I'm with someone I'm crazy about, who I totally enjoy being with, this other way of "overlaying" a fantasy enhances what I have instead of trying to replace it. It's as though your lover momentarily becomes a blend of who they are and the scene you're imagining. The fantasy persona is woven into the lovemaking.

If you're both comfortable with indulging the occasional fantasy about someone else, you might offer your partner a special treat: pleasure them while they enjoy a rendezvous with their imaginary lover. Or indulge their fantasy by playing out their sexy scenario with them. Help each other stay in your roles. You may need to remind them, "I'm your swim instructor, not your spouse!"

"ORAL SEX" HORS D'OEUVRES

Just as appetizers are served to stimulate the desire for dinner, intimate conversations can stimulate the desire for sex. Whether you're making a meal, taking a walk, or just running errands together, "oral sex" gives everyday activities an erotic charge.

There's no pressure to start all the conversations we suggest. You wouldn't go to a restaurant and order every appetizer on the menu. Simply scan through the list and choose topics that interest you both.

Some of these intimate conversation starters will intrigue or inspire you, while others might, for now, feel too sensitive or emotionally charged to jump into. Two people can have wildly different feelings about any particular topic. One may be uncomfortable hearing stories about their partner's past lovers, for example, while their partner loves hearing about theirs. So go slowly, allowing each of you to open up in your own time and at your own pace. When you have a safe, accepting space, simply talking about *why* a particular question makes you nervous or excited can be revealing as well as connecting.

Let's begin with some sexy conversation starters about the past.

- **Your early experiences.** What was your first kiss like? If it wasn't a positive experience, how about your first *good* kiss? Do you remember your first French kiss? How about the weirdest kiss you've ever had, the most awkward, or your best kiss ever?

- **Gender conditioning.** When you were growing up, what messages did you receive about what it meant to be a boy or a girl? Were you ever told that you couldn't do something, or should do something, solely because of your gender? In what ways might gender conditioning have influenced your relationships? In what ways might it be influencing them today?

- **Crushes.** What actors, singers, teachers, or athletes did you have a crush on when you were younger? Tell me about the first person you were ever romantically attracted to.

- **Your erotic memories.** What erotic scenes from books or movies do you recall? Do you remember any X-rated photos you saw early on and what you thought about them? What's one of your earliest memories with a sexual component? What other sensual or erotic experiences or memories come to mind from when you were young?

Of course, it's not possible to predict where any of these conversations might lead. Take Jennifer and Jason, who are in their forties. They had been dating a couple of months, and making love for just a few weeks, when Jennifer coyly broached the subject of their earliest erotically charged memories.

Jason hesitated a moment before looking Jennifer lovingly in the eyes and telling her about how embarrassed he used to feel changing in the school locker room when he was a boy. "Oh, why?" Jennifer asked, feeling concern for whatever it was he had suffered through back then. "Well," Jason told her gently, "I wasn't circumcised, but all the other boys were."

Jennifer realized with shock that Jason's hesitation in sharing this story wasn't because of any shame he was still feeling. He was hesitant because he knew that despite Jennifer being quite educated, she was also very inexperienced sexually and hadn't yet realized that he was uncircumcised. "I went right home that night and did some research to understand exactly what I was working with!" she laughs.

As you share your thoughts on any topics like these, always pay attention not only to how you're feeling, but also to your partner's body language and facial expressions, which can give you insight into how *they're* feeling.

- **Fantasies and dreams.** What did you fantasize about when you were a child, a teenager, or a young adult? Do you recall any fantasies or dreams about sex that a friend or lover described to you? Do you remember any sexual dreams you've had?

- **Your early sexual education.** Where did you learn about sex growing up? Did your parents talk about it? Did you have any kind of sexual education classes at school? What silly or crazy ideas did you have about sex? Do you remember any conversations you had with friends? When did you first learn about oral sex or intercourse? What do you recall thinking about sex before you actually experienced it?

- **Sexual language.** What does the word *sex* mean to you? What words do you find sexy (like *kiss*, *wet*, *swollen*, or *stroke*)? Are there any sexual words you feel particularly awkward or excited saying aloud? What terms for genitals do you prefer? Are there any that make you uncomfortable?

- **Self-pleasure.** When did you learn about masturbation? If you've masturbated, did you know about it before trying it or did you discover it on your own? What do you remember about your first few times: the circumstances, how you went about it, and how you felt about it?
- **Previous attractions.** How many times have you been in love? What about in lust? When you think back to the people you've been attracted to over the course of your life, what themes or similarities do you notice?
- **Your various firsts.** What do you recall about any of your "firsts"? Some of your firsts might be the first time you got naked with someone, the first time you touched someone else's breasts or genitals or someone touched yours, the first time you had any oral-genital contact, the first time you really enjoyed sex, the first time you had intercourse, or the first time you experimented with anal play.
- **Your sexual past.** Looking back at your past relationships, how did the intimacy between you and your partners change over time? Is there anything that you regret or would approach differently if you could do it over again? What encounter would you re-experience if you could? Do you recall a time something significant happened when you were making love—like finding out a musician you like had just died or when a police officer knocked on the car window?
- **Your sexual self.** How comfortable with your sexuality do you feel? How do you feel about your genitals? Have your feelings changed over time?
- **Orgasms.** If you experience orgasms, describe how an orgasm feels to you. Do you have different types of orgasms? If you've never or rarely had them, how do you feel about that?

Any of these topics can be very sensitive, depending on someone's personal history and experiences. For example, someone whose first sexual encounter was unpleasant or traumatic, or someone who doesn't experience orgasms, may find that those subjects bring up feelings of fear, frustration, or embarrassment. It's always okay to not talk about any particular topic with your partner, and it can be helpful to speak with a mental health professional if you have distressing memories, worries, or shame around any aspect of sexuality.

On the other hand, if you *do* feel safe speaking with your partner, sharing something deeply personal or that you've been holding back can allow you to experience their love, compassion, and acceptance. This can bring you closer together and be quite healing.

In addition, someone whose experiences have been limited may not have much to say about some of these topics and feel inadequate. If so, they could try looking for ways to view that inexperience from a positive perspective, such as, "I haven't had many 'firsts,' which means I get to experience some of my firsts with you!"

The remaining questions relate to your relationship in particular.

- **Your early relationship.** What were you attracted to in each other when you first met? What do you remember about how your partner looked, felt, smelled, or tasted? What did you like about the way they kissed, touched, or made love? What surprised you, if anything?

- **Romance and turn-ons.** What makes you feel romantic when you're together: candles, firelight, champagne, massage? What articles of clothing, either to wear yourself or to see your lover in, give you an erotic charge, such as stockings, long skirts, or a particular pair of pants? What little things—like neck kisses, ear nibbles, or foot massages—are big turn-ons for you? What makes you feel desired?

- **Your sexual connection.** What do you enjoy most about your sexual connection? What does having a good sexual relationship mean to you? What gets in the way of you being present during sex? How might your sex life be different if you were both completely comfortable with yourselves and your desires?
- **Sexual activity.** Of the sexual activities or positions the two of you enjoy most often, what makes them a turn-on for you? What have the two of you done that stands out or that you'd like to try again? What have you never done, such as fantasies or ideas you had when you first got together, that you might be up for trying? If you put your minds and bodies to the task, how many days in a row do you think you could have sex? (First, of course, you would have to define what exactly counts as "having sex"!) What are the fantasies and desires you'd love to make happen together sooner rather than later, and definitely don't want to miss out on?
- **What if?** Some couples have given each other a free pass for the billion-to-one chance they meet their idol and that person just happens to want to have sex with them. If your partner is ever lucky enough to get lucky with their idol, would you give them a pass? Who would you use *your* pass for?
- **Your sexual energy.** Did you see anything sexy or intriguing today? What's the hottest thing you've thought about this week?
- **Your most recent intimate adventure.** What did you really enjoy about your last adventure together? Were you nervous? Did anything surprise you? Did you get any insights from it?

When you're in the habit of having provocative conversations, you won't be that couple who spends an entire dinner date looking at their phones or only speaking to each other when it's about ordering the food or paying the bill. You'll be the playful couple looking into each other's eyes with a lusty sparkle!

PLAYING WITH DESIRE

We'd like to tell you the story of an intimate adventure of our own that took place in our living room.

We'd been friends with Raven, a professional dancer, for years when she mentioned she'd started performing as a shibari rope model. Shibari is a Japanese style of rope bondage gaining popularity in the West and especially in kink and BDSM circles ("B" stands for bondage, after all). Typically a trained "rigger" or "rope top" ties the "model" or "rope bottom" using specific arrangements of ropes and knots to create wildly varied artistic forms with the model's body. We were excited to hear what Raven found so compelling about this erotic art form.

"I live a very independent life," she explained, "and the process of being tied allows me to fully surrender, to be completely vulnerable and exposed. It's an interpersonal journey and incredibly meditative. My left brain, that self-doubting voice, finally turns off."

Thoroughly intrigued, we asked if there might be a time we could watch one of these sessions. So one evening, Raven brought a friend of hers, a shibari top, to our home and gifted us with a private performance.

While Raven went off to the restroom and we cuddled up together on the couch, Nigel spread a mat out in the center of the wood floor and positioned a pair of speakers and two large cloth bags in the space. He turned on his music, something instrumental and sensual.

Raven entered the room. Dressed only in a pair of lace panties, she knelt down on the mat, closed her eyes, and bowed her head. Lit by the candles we'd placed all around, she looked enchantingly beautiful.

A few moments passed. Nigel reached into one of the bags and drew out a heavy bundle of rope. He took a few steps around Raven, tracing the fingers of his free hand along her shoulders, then let the bundle fall on the floor beside her. The thump of rope against wood reverberated through the room, but Raven remained motionless. He dropped a second coil of rope on her other side.

Nigel knelt behind her, wrapping his arms around her body. They began breathing together, and we could see Raven relaxing with each breath. He inhaled deeply, smelling her ("breathing me," Raven would say later) and tenderly kissed one shoulder, then the other. She melted into him, her hair falling across her face like a veil. With one arm firmly embracing her, he reached for a length of rope. He loosely wound one end around her free arm, pressed it into her flesh, and then pulled so that it uncoiled against her skin. He repeated this motion a few times, tracing the rope across her chest, shoulder, and arm. Finally, he deftly bound her hands and arms behind her back, then spun her slowly around to reveal his intricately tied symmetrical knots.

Over the next hour, we were mesmerized by their intimate dance. As he tied her, the speed, force, and rhythms of his movements varied, conveying emotions from tenderness and warmth to longing and lust. Even as he occasionally untied and retied parts of her into new positions, his body was always in contact with hers. As he pressed himself against her in different ways, sometimes caressing her or squeezing a breast or a thigh to reposition it, she at times sighed or shuddered, but mostly she just flowed with him, completely relaxed and perfectly in sync with his movements. This was a different persona from the vivacious and energetic Raven we knew. Being so close, we could see the intensity and concentration on his face, the utter surrender on hers. Every so often he took her face in his hands, and she'd open her eyes and they would stare deeply into each other.

When the tying was complete, every part of her body was bound in some way, a human sculpture of skin and rope. Nigel now moved parts of her into new shapes, further highlighting her curves, flexibility, softness, and strength.

The profound connection between them continued as he untied the binds. At times he would embrace her, massage a newly freed arm, caress her cheek, or stroke her hair. When he unwound the last rope from her wrists, he cradled her in a long embrace. It was a while before she slowly began to move and sat up to have some water.

The whole experience—from the rope artistry, to the abundant sensuality, to the depth of emotions that were conveyed—created an intimate adventure for us we're unlikely to ever forget. It made such an impression on me (Mali) that I dreamt that night of being a royal courtesan in Japan centuries earlier, observing a performance of erotic bondage from the most coveted seats in the theater.

Watching this moving sensual art also gave us a personal understanding of what attracts Raven, and many others, to this practice. First, she appreciates it as an artistic expression. "I just love the way it looks, the shape of rope," she says. "I'll see pictures later and think, oh, I look beautiful there."

Second, it's intensely intimate. "We're communicating on a deeper level. I have to be sensitive to how he's moving so I can breathe and move with him." He has to listen to her as well: "There's so much nonverbal communication, because if a rope becomes too tight, it can cut off circulation or damage a nerve. It's necessary for me to indicate my discomfort, so I need to be totally quiet in my mind and present in my body. He'll touch me to squeeze his hand so he knows I still have feeling. When I lost feeling one time, he immediately cut all the ropes, even though it takes two hours to prepare them for a session."

It's also extremely meditative, as it takes Raven's unwavering attention to stay relaxed. Most of her sessions involve suspension as well, which requires surrendering to the physical intensity even more. "If you're moving against the harness and ropes, they'll tighten up. They're tied in such a way to force you to relax," Raven says. "It's liberating to have to let go of fear and of being in control. I always feel really happy after I do rope, because my mind is quiet."

Finally, she also enjoys shibari as a multisensory experience. "There's so much sensory intensity: the feeling of the rope, the tightening, the body's positioning." One artist she works with will weave special low-temperature candles into the binds, and then light them. "The wax starts dripping on my skin, and the feeling is amazing! Later he scrapes off the wax with a knife. It's this great sensation. I know he's not going to cut me but it's so right on the edge!"

All of these reasons speak to why many people are drawn to shibari, wax play, and other kink activities: the state of relaxation and presence that's required, the intimacy, and the intensity of the sensations. And it can be deeply fulfilling to be the center of attention, the object of desire.

And what about the role of the "top"? Why would a person be attracted to tying someone up? People have various motivations. There's the art form itself, whether expressed through performances or photographs. There's also the experience of being in complete control. Just as some people feel they're naturally more submissive, other people are naturally more dominant.

"I love being able to give someone an experience where they can totally surrender," says Nigel. "There's so much joy in being the one to help her really let go."

Shibari and other forms of erotic power play are an opportunity for couples to add adventure to their love lives. If you decide to experiment with any kind of power play, make safety your top priority. Raven stresses how essential it is for anyone in a submissive role to advocate for their own well-being. For example, she would only engage with someone who's educated and experienced.

"Rope artists can spend years learning how to tie because so much can go wrong," she says. "They're in control of how much pressure is on your nerves. You're totally in their hands. If an artist wants to try something new, we talk about it: 'I'd like to do this,' they'll ask, 'do you think you'd be up for that?' You should never feel pushed beyond where you want to go."

It may seem ironic, but knowing that the person in the dominant role has your physical, emotional, and sexual well-being in mind is what makes the submissive role so liberating. "You have to feel held in safety to be able to completely turn yourself over to the experience," Raven explains. "It should feel like something you're creating together, not like something being 'done' to you."

There is a huge advantage to exploring these options as a couple—you have each other's backs! If you're interested, you will want to start slowly and build trust over time. There are plenty of excellent resources available, as well as online and in-person communities for sharing information and learning how to practice safely. Educating yourselves, taking classes or workshops together, and going to kink or BDSM events or shops will give you all kinds of exciting ideas to experiment with.

Jolene and Wes have been dabbling in BDSM for a couple of years. "When he commands me to do something, I love it. I don't have to think!" Jolene says. She also loves the feeling of being desired: "Wes taking control makes me feel that he really is here with me, he really wants me." Wes says that power games have helped them let go of habitual ways of relating sexually and break free of always needing to be kind and thoughtful. He also says they're exceptionally bonding: "All it takes is a wink or a look to take us right there. We share a secret life!"

For other couples, BDSM can be a way to knock down defenses they've built up around their sexuality. Donna, for example, likes her partner to spank her once in a while. "I can't explain exactly why, but it's freeing. It helps me let go of my self-judgment and my feelings of shame around my body."

Of people who have explored some form of power play, some have a preference for being dominant or submissive in bed, while others enjoy both roles at different times. The same goes for simply initiating sex. Some people are usually or always the initiators of sexual activity in their relationships, while others rarely or never initiate. If one person must always start things up, even though they too would enjoy being seduced once in a while, their own initiations may eventually start to come from a sense of duty rather than a feeling of desire. As with any area of sexuality, the more versatile you can be, the more varied your experiences together will be. If you're reluctant to be the initiator or to dominate once in a while, taking the lead is an erotic edge for you to explore—especially if it's something your partner would enjoy. Or if you're always the initiator or in the dominant role, being the receiver or surrendering might be an interesting edge for you.

Letitia resisted taking control in the bedroom for a long time, even though her husband Evan periodically mentioned that it's something he would like. Even now, it's not something she does often, but when they're on vacation and have more time, she's actually learned to enjoy it. She describes being on top of him, grinding against him, squeezing and slapping his chest, and taking pleasure from his body.

"Sometimes I'll strap him down, put on that Madonna song, stand over his face, and 'force' him to service me," Letitia laughs. "Why do I do it, even when it's not my thing? Because it's really sexy to see him so turned on!"

TRAVELS IN TIME

Another (fun and romantic!) adventure of ours began when we retrieved our mini rental car in the heart of the city of love. We wove our way out of the frenzied Paris traffic and into the countryside, zipping past green fields and lush forests and through picturesque villages bursting with flowers in every color. Although the white cliffs of Normandy, the Gothic cathedral where I (Joe) lit a candle in memory of my mother, and the lively sidewalk cafes were all highlights, the part of our trip we were anticipating the most was awaiting in a small farmhouse in the French countryside where we were headed next. We'd been invited there by an old friend of Mali's.

An exuberant sheepdog bounded out of the house to greet us, followed by a charming couple, Kevin and Viviane, offering hugs and cheek kisses all around. Dog lover that I am, I spent a few minutes playing with Willis, who I learned had been a gift for Kevin from Viviane. They graciously ushered us inside for champagne and plates filled with local specialties.

Kevin, a chef by profession, had dated Mali decades earlier. It was her first significant relationship, and over those four years she had many formative experiences. When the relationship had run its course, the two of them parted amicably, wishing each other the best as they moved on to the next phases of their lives. They had recently reconnected when Kevin, who had been very close with Mali's mother, had seen the notice of her death and reached out. When the opportunity came for us to visit the country where Kevin and his wife lived, we were very excited.

Relaxing in their beautifully renovated old farmhouse, we talked and laughed for hours. Kevin recalled stories from long ago that Mali had forgotten, and I loved learning more about her and what shaped her into the woman she is today. I also completed a little mission of my own: personally thanking Kevin for teaching Mali how to be creative in the kitchen, a skill I benefit from almost every day. We happily said yes to their invitation the following evening for more champagne and conversation.

When we took our leave that second night, I told Kevin that he felt like a brother to me, and he said he felt the same way. It made perfect sense to me that I would feel such a kinship with this kind-hearted man that Mali had been in love with.

Our time with Viviane and Kevin was a unique experience we'll remember fondly for years to come. Not only did meeting Kevin connect me with a part of Mali's past, but now I'm part of her "Kevin" story too!

Story Time

Another way to connect with each other's pasts and create a shared experience in the present is simply through telling stories about those times. Think about it this way: if your former lovers are off limits, parts of *you* are off limits. You can't talk about how you got to be such a good dancer, or why you love jazz, or that crazy thing you did once. But if you're able to share some of these stories, you and your partner can harness the romantic or erotic energy in those memories for your own enjoyment and pleasure.

Philippe and Lena have been together eleven years. Both have been married before, and they can speak openly about their past relationships.

"He knows that he doesn't have to censor himself with me, that he can be genuine and unarmored about things that are very close to him," Lena says. "Revealing things about his previous loves is an act of intimacy and trust."

"It's a bonding thing for me," says Philippe. "If Lena says, 'Davis and I went to Jamaica,' I think that's nice, Jamaica. But if she says, 'When Davis and I were in Jamaica, we found this deserted beach and had sex on the sand,' that's exciting! There's a way in which I feel like I'm there, and now it's *my* experience too."

For many folks, what Philippe and Lena are describing is just too much. They simply would never want to hear stories about their partner's past sexual experiences or relationships. And that's totally okay.

Cameron and Chris say that talking about prior experiences stirs up sexual energy from the past that they can then enjoy together in the present. "Yes, I do get pangs of jealousy when she talks about her ex-lovers, especially if she had really good sex with them," says Cameron. "But this is the 'hurts so good' kind of jealousy. I *want* to hear about them. When I ask, 'Oh, did you two have a thing?' I *want* her to say yes!"

If you're both interested—and only if you're both interested!—have conversations about what each of you might feel comfortable hearing about, and understand that that may be quite different for each of you. You must also both be okay stopping at any time if one of you starts to feel uncomfortable instead of excited. Then build trust by honoring each other's limits.

Kane will sometimes ask to hear a story about something his girlfriend Heather did before they met, and he'll add, "But not too much detail!" He's not so into the *who* or the *when* as much as he wants to hear about the *what*! "I just want to know what she enjoyed so that I can do that for her—or with her," Kane explains. Heather is more than happy to give him just the details he desires.

If you're telling your partner a story and insecurities surface, be generous with the reassurance. Remind them that you love them and the relationship the two of you have. If you're listening to a story and start to feel anxious, you might tell yourself something like, "Whatever experiences they've had, they're with me now. And those experiences have helped shape them into who they are today." If you've worked with fears and insecurities as a couple, as we explore in chapters 4 and 5, it can be both intimate and healing to look together at what's behind any feelings of discomfort or inadequacy that arise. Also be aware that such feelings can come up later, after there has been time for reflection, even if there was excitement in the moment.

People love a good story—romance novels are a billion-dollar industry. If your partner enjoys hearing sexy stories from your past, such as when you made love to someone for the first time or an unforgettable weekend you went on, make the most of your real-life erotica by stretching the story out and elaborating on the details.

Through sharing our own stories, we've been able to bring the sweetness, romance, and adventure we experienced in the past into our shared present. When I (Mali) was a little girl, for example, I met Alan. His family lived next door to my grandparents, a day's drive from where I lived. Smitten even as toddlers, we got to see each other only once or twice a year.

The summer I was ten, I learned that Alan had a special gift: a beautiful singing voice. He put on Elvis and I sat cross-legged on the floor, mesmerized as he performed song after song for me. That evening at the nearby skating rink, when they lowered the lights for the couples' skate, Alan had requested Elvis's "Can't Help Falling in Love" and sang it softly into my ear as the disco lights twirled around us. I've never listened to that song since without a smile on my face, as I instantly reconnect with those sweet emotions from so long ago. Hearing it with Joe years later, I shared with him the story of my childhood romance. Not only could he feel the sweetness in those memories, but now this has become one of our favorite love songs, too!

Later, in my early teens, I was fortunate to have the experience of making out for hours on end with a boy I really liked, with no rush to take things further. This was a very innocent experience that I think a lot of people miss out on today. Rod had a very particular way of kissing that I've always remembered. When I was telling Joe about it, we decided to try re-creating that kiss—a fun little experiment that had us laughing as much as we were kissing.

I (Joe) know that Mali enjoys hearing about my own youthful escapades, like the time in my early twenties when I was on a slow train through Mexico and met a young German woman and we mutually seduced each other. I was so happy I'd paid the extra pesos for a private sleeping car! Or the time in college when I unsuccessfully tried to talk the friendly twin sisters in my econ class into a threesome. Even though I was shy, they were easy to talk to, and as the night went on I knew I had to give it a shot or I'd forever kick myself. Or during my first job in sales, when the receptionist at one of my regular stops talked me into coming home with her. (Confession: I went pretty willingly!) Every now and then, Mali will ask me to retell these stories, which takes me back to when I was twenty-two and turns me on all over again!

In Memory Of

Some of us may one day find ourselves in a special situation: dating someone who experienced the death of a beloved partner. Depending on how we handle it, we could turn this potentially unsettling circumstance into a connecting one instead.

In this situation, there can be a tendency to want to sidestep the subject or quietly shut down when our partner speaks with fondness of their past love. And yet, if we can remember that every one of us is special, unique, and irreplaceable, we may be able to welcome that person's memory into our lives rather than feeling we're in competition with it. In addition, being able to allow our partner to share their memories with us can be very healing for them and bond the two of us at a deep level.

"I want to know who this woman was, because I love this man and she meant so much to him," says Renee about her boyfriend Andy's wife, whom he took care of for two years before she died. "I don't ever want him to feel he has to hide her memory away." Renee knows from the way Andy speaks of his wife that "he's a good man who enjoys being in a long-term relationship" and that if things keep going the way they have been, she will eventually be a love of his life too. Renee wants Andy to feel comfortable having pictures of his wife out, sharing stories about her, and revisiting special places they enjoyed together.

Kaitlyn lost her first husband to cancer. Over the years, she's shared with her second husband Nathan special moments and photos from her first marriage. "We've even read some of the love letters I received from Darell," says Kaitlyn. "Nathan's there with me when I reconnect with the emotions from those times. Words can't describe how heart-opening this is for me, and for us together."

A Photo Opportunity

Photographs are a potent way to connect with our past. I (Mali) have spent hours with Joe looking at old photos he has and talking about where they were taken, who he's with, and what's happening in the images.

I had my own darkroom in my late teens and twenties and most particularly loved photographing people. Back when I was dating Kevin, I took dozens of portraits of him. Before Joe and I left for France, I sorted through my boxes and found the best of those images to take with us. Whether I would feel comfortable actually bringing them out when the time came, I didn't know.

On the second evening of our visit, Viviane and Kevin told us the story of how they'd met, when they were both traveling the world in their early forties, and how fortunate they felt to have found each other. I felt a strange mixture of happiness and sadness when I spent a few minutes looking through the snapshots on their refrigerator of when they were first together and the day they were married. I was so happy for them and for where Kevin's life had taken him, yet also wistful I hadn't been in closer contact with him to share in the joy of those moments.

I knew Kevin was not one to hold onto unnecessary possessions, and I suspected that Viviane had never seen a picture of him in his twenties. By now, I felt pretty sure she would welcome my sharing those images with her, so I retrieved them from their hiding place inside my handbag.

She carefully took each photo from me as I passed them to her, laying each one in her lap. She couldn't take her eyes off them. These were portraits of her husband taken through the eyes of a woman who loved him.

The last one was the most intimate, a close-up of his face while he was sleeping. She looked at this one for a long time. When she finally looked up, the tears at the corners of her eyes sparkled like tiny diamonds.

I was so happy that Kevin had found such a lovely life partner, and overjoyed that I'd been able to offer her this gift. When I hear about someone urging their significant other to throw away photos of an ex, I will always remember the look of gratitude and love on Viviane's face that extraordinary day.

As studies have shown, having a receptive, adventurous mindset toward intimacy and sexuality is one of the best ways a couple can nurture and sustain passion. Though the time we shared with Viviane and Kevin was not at all sexual, it was certainly intimate, intriguing, and connecting—just the kind of experience that makes our long-term *relationship* feel more like a long-term *adventure*.

Whether you try some of the suggestions in this chapter or are inspired to come up with your own, continue to cultivate your sense of exploration and willingness to play. And commit to saying yes as often as possible!

8

MONOGAMY WITH BENEFITS: PROCEED WITH LOVE

As with everything else in this book, the ideas in this chapter will resonate with some people and not with others. The couples who will be interested in this information are those who are thinking of having—or who are already exploring—some type of intimate experience with another person or persons *as a couple*. We're talking about an intimate adventure that a couple might have together, whether that's once in a while or once in a decade.

This is not an uncommon choice. For example, in a survey of almost 40,000 men and women in happy long-term heterosexual relationships, between 3 and 6 percent of respondents said that they and their partner had had an encounter with a third person within the previous year.[1]

Even though experiences like these aren't for everyone, for some couples they can be another way to bring connection, excitement, and fun into their relationship—as long as those experiences are approached with certain intentions, understandings, and relationship skills in place.

With this in mind, we'd like to offer some guidance for couples considering this relationship option, including

- how to have open, honest, and loving conversations about their readiness for this choice and how they can maintain the integrity of their relationship in the process.
- how to create an environment in which they both feel welcome to voice any apprehensions or concerns, as they know they will be heard and addressed.
- how to compassionately work with the fears, insecurities, or jealousy that can come up when exploring—or even just talking about exploring!—such an intimate edge together.
- how to ensure that their experiences are healthy and positive for everyone involved. Taking others' concerns and desires into account, and ensuring that everyone feels understood and appreciated, is part of what makes such experiences positive and rewarding.

Let's start by hearing from some real couples who are exploring some degree of intimacy with others.

WHEN THE STARS ALIGN

In the stories that follow, you'll see examples of how couples have decided together what kinds of encounters might be right for them. In particular, notice how they support each other through any insecurity or jealousy, as well as how their awareness and intentions help to ensure their experiences are enjoyable for all. And unlike options that are often designed to keep emotional connection to a minimum, such as swinging, sex clubs, or sex parties, notice that these stories involve intimacy on all levels: physical, intellectual/creative, emotional, and even spiritual.

Kensie and Max: An Ongoing State of Possibility

Kensie and Max have been together seven years and have a young son. Like countless others, they feel they are naturally the long-term relationship "type." They enjoy the feeling of belonging, security, companionship, and shared sense of purpose that nurturing a deep connection over time gives them.

From the time they first fell in love, they were both candid about not wanting their relationship to eventually become sexually lifeless, as their prior relationships had. They were also both open to the possibility of, one day, incorporating some type of intimate connection with others into their relationship. They had many conversations about how they might allow for such experiences in their life together in a way that would keep things fresh while also keeping them happily committed to each other.

"We eventually came to the realization that we want to have our sexual adventures together," says Max. "There's just not that much time in our lives. A polyamorous relationship, where we'd each be developing an intimate connection with another person—spending a lot of quality time with them and knowing what's going on in their lives—would require a commitment of so much time and energy. My date night is Tuesday, hers is Thursday, plus alternate Saturdays would leave a lot less space for the two of us. For us, it's better to be able to play with that intimacy and desire within our trusting primary relationship."

Some definitions might be helpful here. *Open relationships* involve having sexual experiences outside the relationship, which may or may not have a romantic component. *Polyamory*, coined in the 1990s from the Greek word *poly* (many) and the Latin word *amor* (love), typically refers to the practice of having more than one romantic loving relationship at a time. The word *polyamory* is also sometimes used by people maintaining multiple, less committed, more casual sexual relationships at once. These are all forms of *consensual nonmonogamy*, meaning that they are created and conducted with the knowledge and consent of everyone involved.[2]

Besides the relative simplicity, Max says that having their experiences together is "more multidimensional than having them separately. I *want* Kensie to be there. Half the intensity is sharing it all with her!"

The couple says that the anticipation of an upcoming adventure keeps them erotically connected in the time leading up to it.

"The ongoing state of possibility gives our relationship a continuous charge," Max says.

"We get to experience the excitement of dating, and we get to do that together," adds Kensie. She says they could spend an entire evening—or several months!—talking about their next encounter, feeling very inventive and turned on together.

"Having someone to explore with and share what you're experiencing is profound," says Max. "There's an exchange of feelings, ideas, and love that grows deeper over time."

Before any encounter with another person, Kensie and Max have the wise practice of collaborating on an explicit intention for the experience, like, "We're here to have a heart-opening time together." Speaking this aloud to each other in advance helps guide their experience and strengthen their connection while the experience is unfolding.

Ryan and Michelle: Dating as a Couple

Ryan and Michelle have been married twelve years and have twin daughters. Eight years into their relationship, they began to have intimate experiences with others once in a while. They call this "dating as a couple." Why is this their preference over having any extramarital experiences separately from each other?

"One word—intimacy!" explains Ryan. "Even if we both had successful outside relationships, it wouldn't necessarily charge up *our* connection. Dating as a couple contributes more to our relationship as a whole. And we have someone to revisit those memories with later."

Does the excitement of being with someone else make the times when it's just the two of them seem dull by comparison?

"Not at all!" Ryan says emphatically. "Of course, there's a 'peak' of excitement when another person is there, but Michelle is always exciting to me. And we have our own peaks together."

"There's a sexual electricity between us all the time, even when nothing out of the ordinary is happening," adds Michelle.

Do they ever feel insecure or jealous?

"There have been times I've started to feel left out or 'less than,'" says Michelle. "But then we all talk about it, and I feel better."

Bringing these feelings up and getting reassurance and love in the moment, she says, is much better than keeping them all to herself. Everyone's *comfort* about what's happening, the couple says, always takes priority over what's happening.

The couple will also communicate later about anything that came up for either of them, whether during an experience or in the days or weeks that follow. Michelle says that this "is one of the ways that knowing others is bringing us to new levels of intimacy."

Ryan says he's had his own moments of insecurity and jealousy when the couple was spending time with another man.

"When he and Michelle were focused on each other, I've suddenly felt like I was on the outside looking in," explains Ryan. "The first time, I tried to just quietly disappear. I discovered through that experience that for me it's super-important to maintain that 'threesome connection' at all times—whether through eye contact or touch or just open communication." He has also learned "to speak up when I'm not feeling included."

So, what kind of relationship structure do Ryan and Michelle feel they have: Open? Polyamorous? Monogamous?

"Even though we occasionally have experiences with other people, our relationship still feels like monogamy to me," Ryan says.

"I'd say we're 99 percent monogamous," laughs Michelle. "And that other 1 percent keeps our entire relationship on fire!"

Victoria and Dawn: Amplifying the Love in the World

Previously both polyamorous, Victoria and Dawn met at a poly event and have been together seven years. After dating for several months, they both realized they weren't drawn to having intimate experiences without the other being present.

"We're still by nature polyamorous, in the most fundamental sense of the word," explains Victoria. "We believe in loving many. We believe in love."

"Our sexual interactions with others are playful in nature but something we take very seriously," says Dawn. "They're a deep expression of love and care and affection and tenderness, in the mix of all the different layers of sexuality."

So why the shift away from "traditional" polyamory, involving separate relationships, to this arrangement, where any intimate experiences they have with others are as a couple?

"A shared experience magnifies everything for me: passion, sensuality, pleasure," explains Dawn. "To be with your lover and be a witness to them having these things is indescribable. When you do it separately, even when you sanction and support each other's other relationships, you're not fully a part of them."

"There's a world of difference between witnessing the authentic experience and hearing about it later," agrees Victoria. "When I'm there with her, seeing the reaction on her face, feeling the energy moving through her, the compersion is off the charts. If she's just telling me about an encounter after the fact, it's more of a description, an interpretation. It will never capture the essence."

The word *compersion* was coined in the 1970s to describe being happy for the romantic or sexual happiness a partner experiences with another person.

When Victoria and Dawn are with a lover and they're all physically engaged with one another, "it's like completing a circuit," says Victoria. "The sexual energy runs through all of us and everything lights up!"

The couple also says that experiencing "NRE" together rather than separately greatly intensifies the sexual or romantic energy between them as well. NRE, or "new relationship energy," refers to the hormone-induced high people often experience when they start seeing someone new. Because Dawn and Victoria are sharing in those heightened feelings, neither of them feels neglected or undervalued, as frequently happens in polyamorous situations when one partner is experiencing the excitement of a new connection and the other is not.

How do they decide whether a particular person or experience is something they want to pursue?

"We're receptive when the circumstances and people feel right," explains Dawn. "With some people, there's an instant, loving connection. Other times we will steer clear of a potential encounter because it isn't as intentional as we're looking for. If something doesn't have a certain amount of depth, it's just not that appealing for us."

"We still have all the positives of polyamory," says Victoria. "It's a gift to have more people in your life who know you intimately, who encourage your growth, who can laugh with you about your quirks and celebrate your successes. And it's just as much of a gift to reflect all of that back to them."

"What we're involved with is a new kind of intimacy," Dawn says. "Sharing what we have with others amplifies the love in the world."

The three couples you've heard from have all expressed some reasons why this "new kind of intimacy" with others might enhance a couple's relationship. But why would someone choose to spend time with a couple?

Nikki: Benefits with Friends

Some people find that having an intimate friendship with a couple is ideal for their current circumstances. This is true for Nikki, a busy single mother. Nikki had dated Dawn several years earlier and developed a friendship with Dawn and Victoria as a couple after the two moved in together. Nikki enjoys having people that she can get together with safely on occasion, to explore and have fun, but with no additional demands on her time and attention.

"A committed relationship wouldn't fit into my life right now," Nikki says. "And I feel no pressure to give them more than I can, because they already have each other."

She says this friendship does wonders for her. They'll make a delicious dinner and then offer her a massage or a warm, sensuous bath.

"It's so lovely to be the center of attention once in a while," she says. "They treat me like a queen!"

Nikki also says that her friends' solid relationship creates a "circle of safety" in which she feels safe to open up and try new things sexually.

In addition, Nikki says, "I like having access to the beauty of who they are as a couple. They're an example of what's possible for me one day when I'm ready for that."

Eliza: Loving Outside the Lines

Another reason someone might be attracted to spending time with a couple is that they have a romantic or sexual interest in more than one gender. Around 5 to 6 percent of women and 1 to 2 percent of men in the U.S. self-report as being bisexual. In addition, around 9 to 17 percent of women and 6 to 8 percent of men say they've had intimate same-sex contact. These figures have been rising as the social stigma around bisexuality (at least in some areas of the world) has been decreasing.

Eliza, a yoga teacher, describes herself as "an empowered female who enjoys both masculine and feminine energy." She met a married couple at a book discussion group. The three enjoyed each other's company and decided to continue their conversation over dinner. Having had both male and female lovers in the past, Eliza says it felt natural when she realized she was attracted to them both and that the attraction felt mutual. Over subsequent dinners, she learned that the two had spent intimate time with someone a few years earlier and were open to that happening again.

Eliza says that as long as she is feeling an "internal yes" to the friendship, and that they're all benefiting from it, she will continue to enjoy spending time with them.

"My experience of myself is expanding through my participation in this trilogy," Eliza explains. "I'm coming to know myself as someone who can love beyond boundaries, and I have a newfound confidence in who I am as a sexual being." She also says that "being seen and celebrated, intellectually, romantically, sensually, and physically, by both male and female doubles the charge."

What is being intimate with them like?

"Everything about my experiences with them is connected," Eliza says. "Sometimes it feels like she is an extension of my feminine energy. Our skin just melts together. There are other times when the three of us become like one. I can't quite tell where my energy stops and theirs starts."

Eliza says that it sometimes feels as if the two of them are energetically connecting through her body. "When I sense their energies coming together through me, it's truly a spiritual experience."

Is she ever concerned about jealousy?

"Through our heartfelt conversations and playful interactions, I now sincerely trust that she gets turned on by seeing my affection with her husband, and how radical and requisite that is. In fact, I *delight* in feeling her response to my attraction to him. I know that I will be invoking something wonderful in her."

The honest and candid conversations they all had up front, Eliza says, were essential for alleviating her initial concerns that becoming more intimate with them might cause some kind of rift in their friendship.

"That depth of communication fosters trust," she says.

What's it like to be the "third" in this arrangement?

The word *third* is sometimes used to describe a person who engages romantically or sexually with a couple. However, this term can sound impersonal and objectifying, and it fails to communicate the importance of *everyone's* thoughts, feelings, preferences, and boundaries being taken into account and respected.

"On one level I know that she's the wife, I'm not the wife. But I'm first in my own way! I feel revered and appreciated for bringing something unique and precious to this trilogy."

Does Eliza have any advice for other potential "unicorns"?

Another term for a person who spends intimate time with a couple, *unicorn* reflects the notion that couples on a quest for someone to join them in the bedroom are searching for something rare—like this legendary, elusive creature.

"One needs to be in a really good place with one's self. I'm able to keep saying yes because I know that I can say no," Eliza advises. "We're all self-aware adults who respect each other and are committed to taking care of ourselves. If something isn't feeling right for any one of us, that will be expressed and explored. It's also important to choose people who are very solid in their connection. If I didn't have trust in their solidity, I couldn't play with them. The love and connection between the two of them makes this possible!"

James: A Full Expression of Sexuality

James, a high school teacher in his forties, is also bisexual.

"I'm a very independent person," he says. "I've never wanted to cohabit with anyone, but I do love having a lot of deep intimacy in my life. So it works for me to have lovers. Not casual sex partners. Lovers."

James has dated three couples over the past several years.

"Given my life and career and how society is, my bisexuality is not something that's had much of a chance to express itself," he says. "The part of me that gets to experience his maleness, and the part of me that gets to enjoy her femininity, are both very strong parts of me. So in this there is a full expression of my sexuality."

James is quick to emphasize that this "isn't just about sex, it's about intimacy. If they wanted me to just be their boy toy, and didn't want me to be a part of their lives in any other way, it wouldn't be nearly as compelling. I want to be able to share aspects of my life with the people I'm hanging out with. It gives the relationship more meaning."

Is there anything challenging about having these types of relationships?

"The hardest part is having to be undercover about it. Because I'm a teacher, I can hardly talk to anyone about this. Most people just don't have a way to understand it. That's sad, because it feels so normal to me."

The isolation and stigma that James feels at being unable to communicate openly about his life and the people who are important to him are not uncommon. Fortunately, more and more people are becoming open-minded about others' orientations and choices around sexuality and relationships.

Does James have any advice for someone considering dating a couple?

"With some couples, it feels like something's lacking," he says. "They're looking to fill in what's missing or to fix something that's wrong. So look for a couple with a high level of integrity, communication, and connection. Choose wisely. There's a world of difference between people who care about you and your experience and those who really don't!"

Where Are *Your* Monogamous Edges?

The stories you've heard so far have all involved a couple and one other person, but there are other forms that shared intimate experiences with others could take. And experiences don't have to involve sex to still be immensely fun and fulfilling.

Just having friendships as a couple with people you can talk frankly about sex with can be entertaining and thought-provoking. So can attending an erotically themed dance, festival, or exhibition together. There is safety and fun in numbers, and you'll have friends to talk about it all with later. As simple as these scenarios are, they are still beyond many people's conceptions of what's okay in a monogamous relationship.

But never mind what *other* people think is okay or not okay. What's vital is that you and your partner thoroughly explore and communicate about where the edges of your *own* ideas of monogamy are. Then you can enjoy the fun of discovering if there are any gray areas in those definitions—gray areas that could potentially be *play* areas! Because every couple's boundaries are different, there's a wide spectrum of possibilities.

There are, for example, couples who enjoy occasional experiences with more than one other person, as in the stories that follow. Unlike typical polyamorous or open relationships, these couples like to have their adventures together, not separately.

Lawrence and Jamar have occasionally traded massages with another couple they met at the gym.

"We're both very tactile people," explains Lawrence. "And we definitely don't mind getting our hands on a couple of muscle boys, something we share an appreciation for!"

Some couples have intimate get-togethers that involve sexual contact, but only between each couple. Brenna and Adam, for example, have spent time with another couple and made love in each other's presence.

"We both have deeply loving relationships, and it's really nice to share that," explains Adam.

"It's so liberating to let myself feel completely at ease in front of other people, people I know and trust," says Brenna. "It encourages me to be more open with Adam, too."

When couples do interact sexually with each other, those experiences can be intimate on other levels as well.

When Madison and Cody decided to experiment with non-monogamy, they attended a couple of group sex events, but found them predictable and impersonal.

"Parties and sex clubs are too much about the sex," says Madison. "They're not about having lovers and being truly intimate."

They've been getting together for two years now with another couple they met on a dating app for people in open relationships. They make dinner, catch up on each other's lives, laugh, dance, and "create some sexual magic together," says Madison.

"Who's to say we don't have a successful marriage?" Cody asks. "We've found a way to indulge our desires for extramarital intimacy without doing it on the sly and running the risk of blowing up our relationship. Doing this together makes our relationship not only successful, but spectacular!"

For several years, Jon and Julie went to swingers' events every few months. Eventually, though, they began to long for more connection in their intimate interactions with others.

"I'm at a place in my life where it's not just about sex anymore," explains Jon.

"I can no longer compartmentalize sex," agrees Julie. "It has to be in there together with love and caring and emotional connection."

The couple began to develop closer friendships with some of the people they'd met at the play parties they had attended.

"Our get-togethers are very intimate, even though we only see each other once in a while," says Julie. "And because there's more safety with people you know well, we're able to go deeper physically and emotionally—as well as creatively!"

A Couple of Caveats

This is probably a good time to mention that lots of folks, including some therapists, often feel negatively toward relationships that are not 100 percent monogamous. They may even believe that any such relationship is doomed to end. Such attitudes can make couples feel like they're wrong or immoral for even talking about such possibilities. Fortunately, there is a growing number of organizations and groups for people in unconventional relationships, and mental health professionals are increasingly receiving training for working with people in alternative relationship styles.

Also, advocates of open relationships sometimes caution against the kind of experiences that we've been talking about because of something known as "couple privilege." This refers to the tendency of some couples—typically a heterosexual couple seeking the company of a bisexual woman—to approach the prospect focused entirely on what they want from the encounter or relationship, with little consideration for that third person's needs or desires. Their attitude is very objectifying. They project their desires and expectations onto a potential play partner and don't truly see or respect them.

With these caveats in mind, for couples who love and trust each other and are at that threshold where they want to explore something that involves others in some way, an occasional intimate encounter with another person or persons might be a good choice. That's if (and this is a big if) those experiences are approached with healthy mindsets, clear intentions, and solid relational skills.

In light of this, the next section explores in detail how partners can help ensure they have each other's backs—and each other's hearts!—so that they grow even more connected through any adult adventures they might have. Just as importantly, couples will discover how best to make all their experiences positive and rewarding for everyone.

HOLD ON TO YOUR KEYS

If you as a couple decide to explore any kind of intimacy with others, our recommendation is to always have your keys with you. No, we don't mean your house keys. We're talking about those six keys to connected sexuality from chapter 2:

- connection,
- communication ("oral sex"),
- trust,
- acceptance,
- mutual support, and
- gratitude.

If this sounds like a lot of keys to keep track of, don't worry. As they appear again and again in the upcoming examples and stories, you'll get a sense of what's necessary to make such experiences enjoyable and beneficial for everyone.

Let's start with the concept that connection comes first. Whatever the two of you eventually choose to do, approach it in a way that will truly strengthen your bond. (This doesn't mean neglecting or disregarding other people you interact with. Feeling connected applies to them as well, as you'll see in the upcoming section "The Golden Rules of Engaging.") Just like when traveling, it's a smart idea to have a plan for how you'll reconnect if you find yourselves apart. The discussion scenarios that follow will help you create a roadmap back to each other in the event you get a little off track. By exploring these hypothetical situations, you'll not only discover what adventures might be right for the two of you, you'll also be able to uncover and even address in advance some of the insecurities or fears that could be stirred up in the process.

Before you start discussing these scenarios together, we strongly encourage you to have already explored many of the conversations we suggest earlier, including the "Intimacy Inquiry" questions in chapter 1 and the topics for "oral sex" in chapters 2 and 8. Those initial conversations will help you decide what you might be ready for and whether other aspects of your intimacy need attention. It would also be helpful to review the suggestions in chapter 3 for creating a non-judgmental space for sharing your interests and fantasies.

Be very honest with yourselves about whether you sincerely believe that you will be able to talk about the challenging emotions that are very likely to arise if you step outside your comfort zones and other people are involved. Intimacy with others may not be a good choice for your relationship if any of the following apply:

- Your partner has disregarded or been dismissive of your feelings in the past.
- You don't feel confident that you'll be able to speak up and advocate for yourself if you're feeling disconnected or something challenging comes up for you.
- You have a feeling that your partner is just seeking distraction or sexual kicks while your primary interest is in deepening your connection with your partner.

All of these are big warning signs that are dangerous to ignore!

Finally, it's important that you both understand that your edges and boundaries around the prospect of intimacy with others are likely to be different. For some people, watching their partner make out with someone else would be easy or even a turn-on. For others, just the thought of their partner being attracted to someone else can bring on strong feelings of anxiety and jealousy.

Exploring Your Comfort—and Discomfort—Zones

When you're both ready, talk about the following scenarios together, each of you answering the questions from your own perspective. When you come to an idea that brings up fear, anxiety, jealousy, or any other strong emotion for either of you, stay with that topic until you've reached a good level of understanding and the emotional space between you feels calm and loving. If it's your partner who's feeling uncomfortable, you might ask questions like, *How would you describe what you're feeling—anxious, nervous, jealous? What thoughts or fears come up for you? Does it bring up a memory or incident from your past? Can you put into words what you might be afraid of or nervous about?* You might also revisit the tools for healing in chapters 4 and 5 and for taking charge of and dissolving jealousy in chapter 6.

- **Scenario 1.** Suppose the two of you are chatting with someone you've just met and you realize that your partner is quite attracted to them. How do you imagine you would feel—uneasy, curious, intrigued? What thoughts might be going through your head? Can you envision the conversation the two of you will have later? Now imagine that you and your partner are talking to someone new and it's *you* who is feeling an attraction. How do you feel—apprehensive, flustered, excited? You look over at your partner and realize that they know what's going on for you. How does *that* make you feel? What would it take to make these experiences feel good to both of you?

- **Scenario 2.** How would you feel if you were out at a club and saw your partner having fun dancing with someone else? What if the situation were reversed and it was you dancing with someone else? In each situation, is there anything either of you could do or say to make this feel more comfortable, safe, or enjoyable for you both?

- **Scenario 3.** What thoughts or emotions might surface if one of you had a flirtatious interaction while you were out together? What would it take for you to both feel secure, happy, and included?

- **Scenario 4.** What thoughts or emotions might come up if your partner were to kiss someone in your presence? Does the image bring up any nervousness, apprehension, or jealousy? If so, what might you be nervous about or afraid of? What might it take for this scenario to feel comfortable or even exciting for you? What would the circumstances be, and what would the two of you have talked about beforehand? Now, from the other perspective, how might it feel for *you* to kiss someone in your partner's presence?

Remember that your purpose for talking through all of this is to consciously increase your intimacy by exploring ideas and growing together. Your verbal explorations might even lead to a powerful new sexual experience with each other. However, if one of you is actually just intent on trying to make something in particular happen with a third person, this won't be the connecting and potentially healing opportunity it could otherwise be—and could very well result in *dis*connection rather than *greater* connection.

As you discuss these possibilities, you might discover something inside your comfort zones that you'd both like to make happen in actuality. Be prepared, though, for the reality to turn out quite different from what you imagined. An unexpected memory or emotion can be triggered in the moment, and something you both thought would be sexy and fun could wind up being upsetting instead. Which means you have more to talk about and more to learn about yourself and each other!

If you'd like to try something that involves some kind of intimate connection with another person but your partner is adamantly against it, it would be wise to consider the following questions: *How important is this to me? What is my interest in it—what am I seeking to get from it? Can I fulfill this desire within my relationship, even to some small degree, in a way that my partner would also be interested in?*

It's perfectly fine if you don't discover anything you both feel excited to try in reality. Just talking about hypothetical future possibilities, and tiptoeing up to your "just enough jealousy" edges, can keep you both energized for a long time! You might even find that the unfolding conversations are more than enough to add new elements to your sexual relationship and that the desire to actually experience another person dissolves for both of you.

From Fantasy to Reality: Awareness, Intentions, and Boundaries

If you do decide to try something out, take it slowly. A big part of any adventure is the anticipation and preparation leading up to it. As part of that preparation, keep using that communication key: *How can we go into this with as much love and awareness as possible? What can we do to maintain our connection the whole time? What if something unexpected comes up for one of us?*

If the two of you have already had an experience with another person or persons, reflecting on that together can give you valuable insights too: *How did that experience go? Could we have gone into it more consciously than we did? Did we all talk up front about our concerns, desires, preferences, and boundaries? Did we have a conversation about our sexual health and safer-sex practices? Did we talk about whether we'd be open to encounters in the future or an emotional connection? Did we create an environment where it was perfectly okay for nothing in particular to happen?*

An invaluable practice for maintaining your connection during any new experience is setting an intention together, like Kenzie and Max do. Here are some examples: "Our intention is to feel our connection throughout the evening, in as many ways as we can." "We're here to enjoy the fun and excitement of getting to know someone new together." "Our goal is to experience as much intimacy and love as possible." By creating a statement of your purpose, you ensure that you're in alignment about why you're doing what you're doing. You'll find that an intention playing in the background will help set the tone for your experience. And if either of you starts to feel insecure or uncertain, your shared intention will also be a reminder of why you're pursuing this experience in the first place and help you decide whether you need to change course.

Even though you might both be enthusiastic going in, involving another person might bring up difficult emotions in one or both of you—if not immediately, then eventually. That's one reason we've offered so many ideas in this book for supporting each other in addressing anxiety, insecurities, fears, and jealousy, and why we recommend that you've already tried some of those ideas and feel confident about your ability to stay connected when these emotions arise.

Before you embark on an experience with another person, plan out how you will support each other if one of you is feeling insecure, inadequate, jealous, or left out. Reassure each other that you're always available: "If at any point you're feeling disconnected, I want to know. If you start to feel nervous, I'm here for you!" Make an agreement that you'll both stay aware of how the other seems to be doing. If you sense that your lover is withdrawing or pulling away, check in. Anytime is a good time to ask, "How is this feeling for you?" Over time, you'll develop trust that you'll be there to help each other identify and dispel fears and insecurities when they arise.

Also agree that if at any point you start to feel disconnected, you'll do your best to speak up. It can be hard to admit to feeling left out, insecure, or jealous in the moment because we don't want to spoil the fun or interrupt what's happening. But these feelings can be doorways into deeper intimacy, so don't miss that opportunity!

Especially if you're someone who has doubted or ignored your own emotions in the past in order to please someone else, know that any feelings you're having are valid and deserve you and your partner's attention. You're more likely to get the reassurance you need, and back to connection, by sharing what's happening for you rather than by trying to stuff down your feelings, play it cool, or power through. Give yourselves permission in advance to say at any time: "This feels a little challenging. I'd love to just relax for a while and reconnect." If you're not feeling connected, your partner will feel that lack of connection too—if not now, then certainly later when you *do* finally reveal what was happening for you. It's also best to speak up early rather than waiting until you're feeling overwhelmed or shut down.

A word of warning. When one person isn't committed to helping the other's experience be the best it can be, they may try to ignore any fears or emotions coming up for their partner. If you can't be counted on to be there for each other, your intimate explorations won't just be mutually unsatisfying. They will also become a source of frustration, heartache, and resentment. One way to gauge your mutual readiness is to reflect on whether the two of you are solid, considerate, and empathetic in the other aspects of your relationship.

Let's return to that point of taking it slow. Suppose Andrea and Desean fantasize together about having an experience with another woman one day. Andrea, however, is not ready to take their idea beyond the fantasy realm. She has a habit of comparing herself to other women and feeling insecure, and she's worried that tendency could turn any such adventure into a disaster.

Whether the couple ever pursues this possibility in real life, they could still have a very intimate time finding ways to address Andrea's feelings of deficiency. For example, by putting themselves in situations that start to activate her insecurity—such as going out people-watching or viewing erotica with a "threesome" theme—they could experiment with many of the earlier ideas for lessening insecurities and discover which are effective for her. Or they could role-play having a conversation with a potential lover in which the three of them come up with a strategy for what to do if Andrea starts to feel uncomfortable. This shared-fantasy experience could be very healing, helping Andrea to quiet the habitual thoughts that make her feel insecure. It could also be very connecting, as it's so rewarding to help someone you love make progress toward letting go of a personal limitation and feel better about who they are.

Or suppose Andrea and Desean have fantasized about getting together with another man, but because of a previous traumatic experience with a cheating spouse, Desean gets anxious whenever they start talking about the possibility of making this fantasy a reality. One place to begin might be for Desean to just observe Andrea having a conversation with another man when they're out at a restaurant or club. Of course, Andrea will want to stay very sensitive to how Desean responds to this experimentation and be there to reassure him that she is 100 percent there to have fun and explore with *him*—Desean—and that they can shift gears or leave at any moment. If this little experiment goes well, Desean might watch Andrea dance with or hug someone else.

The idea here is to generate just a quiver of jealousy or nervousness, only to the point that Desean's antennas start to go up. Then, as described in "The 'Just Enough Jealousy' Edge" in chapter 6, they can take the energy they stir up home and have a fabulous time with it. By soothing any fear or insecurity that might come up for Desean, they can both enjoy the bounty buried beneath his jealousy: excitement, passion, and red-hot desire for Andrea! If Desean finds that he's still having to work with feelings of suspicion or withdrawal, however, that's an indication that the couple should keep the prospect of being with another man as a shared fantasy, at least for now.

Whenever you set agreements or boundaries, honor them. For example, suppose you attend an erotic party with an agreement to stay together and just observe. Don't let impatience or arousal seduce you into getting swept up in the moment and jumping beyond your agreements. If, over time, your lover grows to trust that you won't try to push them past what they're ready for, they'll feel much freer to experiment and play with you.

It's wise not to expand your boundaries in the heat of the moment so that you don't do something you later wish you hadn't. (Going beyond established boundaries tends to happen more frequently when alcohol or drugs are involved, so staying sober is a smart choice.) That said, couples who have developed a loving, accepting environment for expressing whatever they're feeling, and who are always there to support each other, might be perfectly at ease not deciding everything they will or won't do ahead of time.

For us personally—because we can talk about anything, we take every step together, and we're there for each other no matter what—what we have feels quite collaborative in the moment. We say things like, "I'm feeling really good about this and this, not quite sure about that, and definitely not up for *that*." We can honor our edges while simultaneously exploring them. They become a place to play. We don't feel deprived if we stick to playing just this side of a particular line. As we hold these lines, trust builds, until we're both ready to smooth them over and redraw them a little further out.

We want to emphasize again that this works for us because we both feel completely supported by the other. You want to keep yourself safe by trusting what your intuition is trying to tell you, especially if any of these red flags are flying:

- You're feeling confused by your partner's behavior or their words don't align with their actions.
- It feels like your partner isn't concerned about your feelings or doesn't really want to strengthen your connection but just wants to get their way or make something specific happen.
- Your partner is rushing you or you're feeling pushed or coerced into doing something you're not ready for.

- Your partner doesn't want or isn't able to talk about these kinds of observations with you, or promises they will change and then quickly reverts to the same behavior.

If any of this is happening in your relationship, the kinds of experiences we've been talking about in this chapter are most assuredly not advisable!

And what if two people are in complete alignment and mutually supportive but—on one occasion—a trust is broken or a boundary is trampled over? One secret of successful long-term relationships is the ability to forgive. We're all human, and we're all going to mess up sometimes. A couple's connection can actually be strengthened through the difficult but potentially heart-opening process of working together to overcome a misunderstanding or actual dishonesty. This requires vulnerability and self-examination from both people—and often a good counselor—to create an environment of acceptance in which they can disclose and heal their feelings of hurt, disappointment, anger, guilt, and blame and rebuild a stronger foundation. People *can* learn from their mistakes, and a broken trust is sometimes the wake-up call they need to do so. (Note that we specified "on one occasion." Repeated behavior that tramples established boundaries is never okay. There are people who will make endless excuses for their bad behavior, blaming their partner for having concerns rather than taking responsibility for their own actions. That's a relationship someone needs to get out of—not behavior that should be forgiven.)

Experiences with others, even just once in a while, can inspire intriguing conversations about what you enjoyed, what surprised you, and what you might do differently in the future. Use your explorations together to keep the sexy dialogue going: *What were the most romantic or exciting parts of this experience for you? Has this given you any other inspiration or insights? What might we do if we wanted to expand on this one day?*

The final key on your ring is the shiny golden one: the gratitude key. After any experience with others, take some sweet one-on-one time to reconnect and reflect on your latest adventure together. Acknowledge your lover for being on this intimate journey with you. There's a lot to be grateful for when you're with someone who's willing to explore and expand to keep your connection fully alive!

THE GOLDEN RULES OF ENGAGING

The keys to connected sexuality apply not just to the two of you, but to any other people you're planning to be intimate with. Here are some suggestions to help ensure that your experiences are positive and enjoyable for everyone:

Treat any intimate friends as honored guests in your lives. Do your very best to make sure they feel respected and valued. Endeavor to accept them for exactly who they are. It's a unique individual who wants to explore intimacy with a couple, so appreciate the fact that they're choosing to spend time with you!

Leave any expectations at the door. Go into every encounter with a minimum of expectations. This includes having no agenda for what you want your guests to do or who you expect them to be. An open mind will make it much easier to come together and create something loving, exciting, and fulfilling for all of you. If you do have specific ideas about things you'd like to experience, hold them lightly enough that you don't subtly (or overtly!) attempt to manipulate or pressure others or end up feeling disappointed if your wishes don't happen to play out. With no end goals in mind, you'll be much more present with whatever *is* happening.

Time with intimate friends doesn't have to involve specific sexual activities to be both fun and rewarding. Jon and Julie have this to say about the gatherings they host from time to time: "When we get together with our circle of intimate friends, there's always a possibility that something very unique and connecting will happen. At the same time, nothing in particular has to happen. Being with them, no matter what happens, feels juicy, erotic, and packed with potential."

Share your desires, interests, and boundaries. Before any intimate encounter, give everyone an opportunity to share any interests or desires they have, what they're definitely not up for, and what they *might* be up for: "I'm not sure I'll be interested in X or Y, but if everything feels right, I reserve the option to change my mind!" Also make time for everyone to express any concerns or nervousness, like "Even if I don't get hard, I'll still be having a great time!" or "I'm worried you will be disappointed if we don't do Z." Talking about these things up front will take the pressure off and make it easier for everyone to speak up if at any point they start feeling uncomfortable.

If there might be sexual contact involved, be sure to have a conversation about sexual health, including any STIs (sexually transmitted infections), treatments, and recent testing. Talk about safer-sex practices and what you will do to protect everyone's health as much as possible. People often avoid these topics because they can feel awkward. Talking candidly about sexual health, despite any awkwardness, communicates that you are thoughtful and trustworthy and can even increase connection and intimacy.

Discover where your desires align. By creating a safe, agenda-free environment, you make the space for *possibility*. Together, you'll now be able to see where your desires overlap—your shared playspace—and maybe even some interesting edges to play at. Through these conversations, it can seem almost magical how the things in your overlapping comfort zones come into focus and activities or explorations that would be fun, sexy, or sensual for everyone just seem to suggest themselves. Collectively, you might come up with creative ideas that no one would have thought of on their own.

There might be a few surprises in your shared interests, too. It's easier to fulfill some desires when you have the enthusiasm and creativity of more people! A four- or six-handed massage can be a delightful experience, and possibilities for role-playing expand greatly. And being seen and accepted by multiple people at once can be powerful in helping someone let go of a fear or inhibition. Casey, who's been working on not being self-conscious about facial expressions during sex, says that being able to totally let go in the presence of not only her loving partner but another couple as well "means I'm *really* not holding back!"

What if the only thing in your shared playspace is hanging out on the patio in the moonlight in your sexy attire and enjoying a meal together? Then make the most of it! Luxuriate in the sensuality of being outdoors: the smell of the evening air, the sounds of nature, the feel of the breeze on your skin. Savor the textures and the flavors of the food. This is also a perfect opportunity to propose some of the "oral sex" topics in this book as stimulating conversation starters.

Talk about how you can all help ensure that everyone feels fully involved through the entire experience. Any exploration of intimacy among more than two people may naturally become an exploration between just two of them at times. Acknowledge this fact up front, and give everyone the green light to speak up any time they're feeling left out. Talk about ways you might reestablish a feeling of connection if this occurs, such as through eye contact, touch, or speaking with one another.

Everyone needs to do their best to remain aware of the others. If you sense someone pulling away or shutting down, checking in and asking how they're doing can help restore the sense of connection among you. Some people will be very comfortable with others exploring while they are more on the sidelines, while other people won't be comfortable at all. Sometimes you don't know how you'll feel until the time comes. If you're feeling neglected, you might say something like, "I'm feeling a little left out. How about we try some more of that Australian honey kissing we were doing a few minutes ago?"

If you're feeling pretty comfortable and would rather not interrupt what's happening between your "playmates," here are other ways to get back to a feeling of connection. First, remind yourself that just because your partner is experiencing something new and different doesn't mean that what they're experiencing is better. For example, there's something unique about the kiss between any two people. That uniqueness doesn't make it better, just different. Second, try "trading up" what you're telling yourself. Instead of "My partner will want this all the time now" try "I love that we've created an environment where my lover can experience this different way of kissing" or "When I get my lover alone again, *we're* going to kiss like that!" These first two suggestions involve self-soothing your feelings of insecurity, which will allow you to reengage with the activity. Third, lie back and take in the visuals of your partners-in-pleasure enjoying themselves, like the beauty of one person's hands against the other's skin. Fourth, reach out to make physical contact, maybe running your fingertips along the contours of their bodies. Finally, enjoy the feeling of the erotic energy that's being stirred up and perhaps even touch your own body in a way that turns you on.

As it's also natural for there to be different degrees of romantic or sexual electricity between any two of you at various moments, these are helpful approaches to have. With practice, you might even learn to "ride" each other's excitement and feel into each other's feelings and sensations.

Check back in after you and your guests have had time to reflect. Give everyone the opportunity to talk about any thoughts or emotions that came up afterwards or realizations you or your guests have had since. When everyone feels cared for and appreciated, you might even find yourselves dreaming up ideas for your *next* encounter!

OUR TURN

The two of us have shared just a handful of sensual adventures with others over the years. What is our motivation for having experiences like these? We've experimented enough to know that, at least for us, sex parties and clubs are too focused on sex, and too lacking in the other dimensions of intimacy and connection, to hold our interest. And pursuing romantic or sexual experiences with other people separately from each other, as couples in open relationships often do, doesn't appeal to either of us.

Essentially, the handful of encounters we've had with other people are shared experiences of what is so compelling about dating and intimate relationships. We're sharing in that exciting sense of anticipation and fun of getting to know someone new, as well as in any discoveries we make in the process.

In our experiences with others, the focus is always more on intimacy than on sexuality. Even when there's no sex involved (at least none that meets the usual definitions of sex!), these occasions are filled with sensuality, affection, and fun. Some of our most memorable times have involved taking many of the ideas we've covered in this book into an encounter with another person or persons—from exploring the various dimensions of sexual connection, to channeling the energy of jealousy, to supporting each other's growth and healing. Through these experiences, we've learned that the foundation of love, trust, and understanding that two people can create over time can feel so solid and secure that it becomes a "zone of safety" in which others feel comfortable not only being themselves but also discovering new things about themselves.

As so much of what we teach involves healing through intimate connection, it makes sense that there's a healing aspect to every encounter we've had with others—at least for one of us, and often for all of us. Everyone has their personal challenges around sex and intimacy, from insecurities and self-consciousness to areas of fear, shame, and embarrassment. To us, experiences that help someone let go of a self-doubt, break free of a limitation, or explore an interest or desire are fun, intimate, and immensely worthwhile.

A few years ago, while away on a short writing retreat, we met a woman who was around our age. Over a long dinner on an outdoor deck overlooking a lovely valley, Hanna talked about her experiences with intimate relationships. They had been fairly limited and mostly with inattentive, abusive partners. She was very curious about the kind of connected relationship we were describing and asked many questions about what someone would have to know to create such a partnership. From all she told us, and the questions she was asking, it became clear that Hanna had a real longing for intimacy. Eventually she confessed that she had never felt safe enough with a man to even just relax into his arms and be held.

As we began gathering our things to go, I (Joe) asked Hanna if she would like a hug. She glanced over at Mali, who gave her blessing with a smile, and then moved into my arms. She rested her head against my chest. As I held her, Hanna breathed deeply, like she was taking it all in. I felt her let go a little more with each breath. She really did seem to be melting into my embrace.

While this was happening, I (Mali) looked up at the moon through the trees over the deck. I knew that by my presence, I was vouching for Joe, that he was a safe man. Given her past, Hanna certainly needed to know she was with someone safe. When the two of them let go of each other, Hanna and I hugged too.

Before she left, Hanna thanked us for the conversation, and the hugs. She didn't need to thank us. We had both been quite moved by the experience!

The next day, Hanna came across us in one of our favorite writing spots, on beach towels spread out on a grassy hill along one of the main paths. She asked if she could sit with us for a while. She said the energy from the previous evening was still with her, and that she'd never before experienced a hug with a man that lasted long enough that she could actually feel an intimate connection through it.

Hanna asked me how I had felt about them sharing such a long embrace. I said I wished more people had that chance. And that I hoped that one day she would meet someone with the potential for that depth of connection.

Knowing we wanted to get back to our writing, she shyly asked if she could have another hug. As she and Joe came together in their second embrace, I stretched out on my towel, taking in the beautiful afternoon. It was a satisfying feeling to know that through our interactions, Hanna's next choice of a romantic partner might be a much better one.

We saw Hanna just once more, late that evening. She said she'd spent the afternoon taking a long walk and writing in her journal, reflecting on her own unsatisfying relationships and pondering the possibility of meeting someone with whom she could have a far deeper level of connection. Then she told us that only because she was leaving to fly home in the morning did she have the courage to say something to us she'd been thinking about all day.

"I've been wondering," she said quietly, "what it would be like to kiss someone with that kind of caring and presence."

We both had to laugh at the mischievous little smile on her face. We expressed our sadness that she'd never experienced a kiss like that—and how happy we'd be for her to have the opportunity, if she'd like.

As Hanna leaned in toward me (Joe), my intention was clear in my mind: to help Hanna know herself as worthy and desirable and to allow her to experience what could be possible for her. I embraced her as I had before, in no rush, and let her initiate the kiss. At first she held her mouth quite firmly, almost stiff, and the kiss felt tight and unyielding. I gently backed away for a moment and suggested she just let go of any thoughts she was having. After a few moments, her body relaxed and she kissed me again.

As we separated, she held my gaze. Then she said, "I have never kissed like that before. Ever."

Her words made me tear up. Mali and I had kissed that way for so many years. To be the one to kiss Hanna with tenderness and care for the very first time was a real privilege.

For my part, I (Mali) want to address those who might think that Joe's experience with Hanna took something away from us. I'm here to say that just the opposite is true. Helping Hanna on her journey to heal the mistaken belief that she doesn't deserve real love or affection—a potentially life-changing experience for her—was profoundly gratifying for both of us.

More recently, while seeking out new connections with interesting people, we made the online acquaintance of a man named Rick. We were soon messaging back and forth about topics like tantric spirituality, mysticism, and Eastern wisdom traditions as they relate to sexuality—topics we don't know much about.

When we eventually decided to move our conversation to a video chat, Rick spoke passionately about his interest in Hinduism's concepts of the "divine feminine" and "divine masculine." He talked about this not as related to sex or gender, but in a more universal way, much like the principal of yin and yang. The idea of masculine and feminine energy feels similar, in that everyone has access to these energies and can benefit from developing them.

"The divine feminine and masculine energies," Rick explained, "work together. The masculine is the stable, grounding force that provides the supportive foundation for the dynamic, creative energy of the feminine to fully express itself."

I (Mali) have always considered myself in touch with both my masculine and feminine sides, or my yin and yang qualities, as Joe and I wrote about in our book *The Soulmate Lover*. It's unfortunate that there is such gendered language for these concepts. Without that, it would be much easier for many people—including me!—to explore the underlying ideas that there are many different and valuable aspects of being human and that everyone can develop and benefit from them.

Gendered language aside, Rick's take on these concepts intrigued me, especially given that the recent impacts of menopause and the isolation of the Covid-19 pandemic had left me feeling low-spirited and lethargic where my libido was concerned. The abundant sexual energy that has always been such a creative force in my life felt like it had cooled to a low simmer. Here we were just about to finish a book on ways to keep the passion in a long-term relationship alive and I was feeling, quite uncharacteristically, not very passionate at all.

I admitted to Rick that I currently felt disconnected from that "dynamic, creative energy of the feminine" he was speaking about. It occurred to me to ask how he thought I might start renewing that energy and get my sexual mojo back.

Rick, a massage therapist, replied that he believed physical touch and intention could be helpful. "Through loving, no-agenda touch," he said, "grounded masculine energy can be run through the hands to activate feminine energy in someone else and assist it to flow."

"Well, *that* sounds fabulous," I said.

"I've only done this with lovers before," Rick said, "but I believe this is something that Joe and I could do for you."

Intrigued, I looked over at Joe. "I'm certainly open to learning how to do that," he said to me. "I'm willing if you are!"

Who was I to say no to such an offer—especially one brought to me through the hands of two sincere, warmhearted men? Besides, if there's one thing I love, it's an intimate adventure!

We lived several hours apart, so the date we arranged was a few weeks away. In the meantime, Rick suggested I choose some relaxing music for the experience. This may sound crazy, but listening to music for relaxation was something I'd never done. I enjoyed experimenting, playing various pieces and asking myself: *Does this make me feel relaxed? How about this?* This friendship was already bringing new things into our lives and we hadn't even met in person yet.

Over dinner the night Rick arrived in town, we got to know him as a genuine and intelligent person. We both felt comfortable around him and were excited for the experience to come.

But when he returned the following evening, we didn't get right to the massage. Instead, Rick asked if we had cushions to set around the low table in our living room. On the table he arranged a teapot, cups, and the traditional accessories to perform a Chinese *gungfu* tea ceremony. We took our places on the cushions. As the water was heating, Rick talked about the ceremony.

"To me, taking time for ritual in relationships is important," he began. "Our relationships are so often dominated by work and children and the household and whatever else must be attended to. Ritual is a way to help us reconnect with the purpose of our relationship independent of those externalities." He spoke slowly, almost meditatively. "The tea ceremony allows us to slow down, to notice, to breathe, to be present together as we share in something ancient and sensual. And the tea-drinking ritual *is* quite sensual. There is a focus on something beyond just drinking: on the senses, on rhythm."

I could tell by his smiling eyes that Joe was feeling as enchanted as I was to be hanging out in our familiar space while a new friend shared their passion and knowledge with us—and as grateful that our relationship allows for, and even encourages, having cool new experiences like this one.

By the time the last tea had been poured, we'd been sitting quite a while. Rick asked if there was anything I needed so that I'd be comfortable lying down for an extended period. I was excited that the event we'd conjured up was finally about to begin, but my body did feel stiff after sitting so long. I said that moving to some music would help loosen me up. We had fun dancing around together to a couple of songs. Well, I probably had the most fun—dancing my heart out with my two handsome dance partners was quite energizing!

It was finally time. Because he knows I get cold easily, Joe had already warmed up the room. I switched to the playlist of soothing music I'd put together as Joe lit several candles and turned off the lights. With the sun going down outside, our living room suddenly felt quite romantic. Then Rick surprised us. He had brought a full-length heating pad for our massage table. When Joe saw my delight at that thoughtful touch, he said he knew just what he was getting me for my upcoming birthday!

While the guys moved the massage table to the center of the room, I stripped out of my clothes. Being fully naked in their presence for those brief moments, I felt playfully mischievous and even somewhat like a goddess. Being the center of attention was quite sexy! I slipped under the sheet they were lifting up for me, lying face down as Rick directed.

Four hands came to rest upon my thighs. Rick started talking softly: "To sense this subtle but powerful energy, one needs to be in a receptive state, to focus inward." Then to me he said, "There is nothing you need to do. There is no expectation of you here. You don't need to serve anybody, or do anything, or experience anything in particular. There is no timeline, no hurry, no agenda. And please speak up if something is not feeling good to you." Then to Joe I heard him say, "We do this without an objective, without any desired experience, with just a love for Mali and her spiritual energy. We'll work together, in unison, through her. We can also talk during this and share what we're experiencing." Finally, he reiterated, "There's no deadline for when this will be over. We're in no hurry. Opening requires time."

Nothing much had happened, yet being directed to not think about having any particular response or reciprocating in any way—that I was just to let go and allow myself to receive—already had me feeling like I was melting into the table.

As the two moved their touch from one area of my body to another, I was aware that they were both there, but often not specifically which pair of hands belonged to which man. I heard Rick talking about holding their palms over certain chakras, or energy centers, or moving their hands in repetitive motions to awaken and guide the energy. I found the experience more relaxing than the deep-tissue and Thai-style massages I'd had in the past. Besides calming down my usually busy mind, having four loving hands caressing my naked body felt absolutely decadent. I eventually turned over and they continued on my front side.

When all four hands finally came to rest on my stomach, Rick quietly asked if I had any special requests before they finished up. Apparently a spark of the sexual energy I'd been missing had been conjured up, as I said something like, "I heard you two mention the passion you share for the female form. How would you feel about massaging me a little longer while focusing on sending that desire you feel through my body?"

The men took no convincing. Together, they began kneading and stroking my entire body while I concentrated on what I was feeling. The sexiness dial on this experience had just been turned up and I undeniably sensed my sensual appetite being charmed into motion. By the time they finished, I felt simultaneously blissed out and sexually charged up, a heavenly combination. I got dressed and we moved outside under the stars to talk.

My companions were quite curious to hear about my experience. Whether it was "divine masculine" energy waking up my "divine feminine" energy or simply that doing something creative and edgy had lit a spark in me, the experiment had had the desired effect. As the three of us chatted, two insights emerged.

First, to keep my sexual energy circulating, I needed to pay more attention to whenever I *did* experience moments of feeling sexy or turned on. And second, Joe and I needed to take our own advice and keep finding ways to expand the edges of our sexual comfort zones. Doing so was essential to help mitigate the effects that anxiety, stress, and getting older might otherwise have on our libidos. Intimate adventures are truly preventative medicine!

Rick had one last thought to share. "Why not see menopause as a metamorphosis into a whole new phase of your sexuality, natural and by design?" he asked. "As a time to just be curious about how your libido wants to express itself now?"

His words were instantly liberating to me. How different it felt not to focus on this time in my life as the loss of something I wanted to get back, but as an exciting new era of my sexuality. I believe this idea could also be helpful for people experiencing dips and changes in their libidos at any stage of life.

Over the next few weeks, I continued to feel that the experience with Joe and Rick had given me a lift out of the sexual doldrums I'd been in. I starting having dreams about sex again, which I hadn't had in what felt like a long time. And when Joe and I attended a wedding a few weeks later, I found myself thoroughly enjoying a fun flirtation with a couple of men there—and sharply aware that the social isolation of life in a pandemic, by keeping interactions with new people to a minimum, had exacerbated that sense of losing my sexual spark.

I wasn't the only one who took something valuable from our time together. After he returned home, Rick told us that being able to share his knowledge and passion in a context where they were welcomed and celebrated had increased his sense of confidence in himself.

And as for me (Joe)? I would describe our time together as a spiritually sexy experience. Or a sexy spiritual experience. Actually, it was both! That's not to say it wasn't initially challenging to consider massaging my naked partner with another man—it was. But knowing that it wasn't going any further than that, and intimately aware of how much Mali enjoys an erotic experience with an edge, it was easy to say yes. I really got the sense that Rick was sincere in his desire to help Mali reconnect with the source of her creative sexual energy, which is such a part of who she is and who she wants to be. And watching her all fired up flirting with those guys at the wedding, I'd have to say I'm really looking forward to seeing what else this new stage has in store for us!

We can't resist sharing one last story with you. Cece is a vivacious woman with whom we'd had a fun, flirtatious friendship for many years. During that time, she had dated several men. They were all friendly, attractive guys, but the relationships never moved beyond casual, even though Cece was definitely interested in finding a connection with long-term potential.

One night she called us with some big news. She'd had a few dates with another great guy—and had just broken it off. But by spending time with him, she said, she finally understood the reason her dating endeavors had never been long-lasting.

"He's the perfect lover, kind and beautiful and fun and attentive, and it still didn't work for me," Cece said. "Everything was there—the trust, the safety, the attraction."

"So what's the problem?" we asked, thoroughly intrigued.

"The thing is," she said slowly, "at my core, I'm a lesbian!"

It had taken thirty years for Cece to realize this about herself, she explained, because of her strict religious upbringing. Embedded deep within her psyche was the belief that "being a lesbian would mean I was going to go to hell. I could never even consider the idea that *that* might possibly be *me*!"

We were thrilled for her, and honored to be witnesses to her remarkable discovery. Later we decided that Cece embarking on a new phase of her life's journey called for a little celebration. I (Mali) remembered our very fun "pussyfest" from years earlier, in which Joe and I had visually explored a few hundred pictures featuring a vast variety of vulvas. As a newly out lesbian, Cece, I thought, might enjoy something similar.

With Joe's enthusiastic assistance, I selected about seventy sensual photos. Cece being the artistic type, I added several more images showcasing jewelry and tattoos, as well as a few vulva paintings, drawings, and sculptures. I also had fun putting together a playlist of songs with just the right sensual feel, including some artists I knew Cece loved.

The next time we got together, we made her wait until after dinner (and several choruses of "No, we're not giving you any hints!") for her surprise.

Propped up by throw pillows, we snuggled close together on our bed. Cece was in the middle, my laptop open on her thighs.

For a moment, it felt slightly awkward to be viewing such erotic images together. Cece then confessed that the idea of being face-to-vulva with someone she was dating might be a challenge. But as we took in one photograph, then another, and another, we all got comfortable, and Cece started to get very excited. She loved the diversity, all the different colors and curves and textures and hairstyles. She was also noticing similarities. Some were shaped like butterflies, while others resembled tulips, hearts, madonnas, or angel wings.

"Every one, every pussy on the planet," she mused aloud, "is an original work of art!"

Cece called us the next day to say that the experience had made her cry and that she would be thinking about it for months.

"I will never forget that healing evening," she said sweetly.

For me (Joe), I have to say that this evening was not only incredibly moving and gratifying, but erotic and fun. As I've already confessed, I am, after all, a confirmed pussy man!

We received another call a few weeks later, the morning after Cece and a woman she'd been dating "finally took their panties off."

Instead of being nervous about getting naked with her, as Cece believed she would have been prior to the vulva celebration, she was excited to see this unique work of art unveiled before her. She says she looked upon it "as a thing of wonder and beauty."

"She is a *madonna*!" Cece informed us, breathless. "She is magnificent!"

Friendships like these offer us what many people in long-term relationships wish they could experience once in a while: the excitement of intimacy, connection, and fun with someone else. We've found a way to get that desire met *together*, within the safe, solid framework of our relationship, and in a way that benefits everyone.

In our relationship, we're not only *allowed* to meet new people and make new and interesting friends, we're *inspired* to. Because we know that through these friendships, we will hear new stories, learn new things, be introduced to new ideas and new ways of thinking—all of which keeps our time together interesting and compelling.

Our experiences with others—many of whom we call our "soul friends"—will continue to have positive effects on us far into the future. We picture ourselves sitting back in our rocking chairs one day, laughing and reminiscing about the exceptional times we've shared and the very special people we've shared them with, and feeling immense gratitude for all the healing, growth, and fun we've had together.

HAND IN HAND

Of all the ideas we've explored in this book, can you guess which is our personal favorite? The answer might surprise you. It's just this: the simple luxury of spending a long sexy weekend alone together.

These weekends are occasions we both look forward to, times

we put aside day-to-day tasks and distractions and settle into the slower pace of our cherished Mali and Joe time. Maybe we go somewhere or maybe we stay at home, but either way we fire up our ever-growing collection of love songs, light a ridiculous number of candles, and let passion and creativity have their way with us. Whether we're enjoying some delicious food, exploring a crazy new idea, or making pleasurable use of some really good chocolate, these are precious opportunities for us to romantically and sexually reconnect.

As our holiday-for-two comes to a close, we laugh together as we return furniture and mirrors to their proper spots and hunt down the lingerie that's been scattered from one end of the place to the other. And we smile knowingly to each other as we contemplate all the sweet and sexy memories we've made—often in every room!

The love high we're on can last for days, and sometimes weeks.

Without a doubt, we can tell you that when it's just the two of us, there's nothing lacking or missing. When it comes to the experiences we've shared with other people, we've never had them because we're bored with each other. In fact, it's just the opposite. We've had those experiences because we're both so excited by all the different aspects of sexuality—connection, sensuality, passion, and, of course, healing and growth. We're never bored. We're just fascinated!

The occasional intimate adventures we've had with others have introduced us to new ideas, interests, and experiences. They've helped us to see each other, and ourselves, from new perspectives. Every interaction we've had has encouraged us to grow—whether that's in self-acceptance, self-knowledge, or self-confidence, or in our understanding and appreciation of one another or someone else. And the memories we share of our encounters are a treasure chest of inspiration for sexy conversations and future possibilities.

Whether we're role-playing a curious extra-terrestrial and its willing captive or dreaming up a sensual, healing evening with a close friend or two, we want to keep having intimate adventures, and we want to keep having them together. Having our adventures together lights up our whole lives! And because what we have is so multi-dimensional and so satisfying on every level, our most compelling sexual interest is, and remains, each other. Our experiences with others are something we cherish, yet if we never had another, we would both be happy to continue making the very most of just the two of us. We're both so grateful to have found in the other a true life partner: someone to enjoy, appreciate, and celebrate everything life has to offer, including all the various realms of sexuality.

We're in complete agreement that walking away from this non-stop intimate adventure we're on is inconceivable. We're also both dedicated—heart, mind, body, and soul—to doing everything we can to keep our crazy sexy love affair going as long as possible.

Afterword: An Invitation

Thank you for joining us on this journey into fueling the erotic in long-term relationships to deepen love and connection. Our heartfelt wish is that you come away from this book excited about all these possibilities for keeping your relationship emotionally, mentally, physically, and even spiritually intimate. And we hope you're feeling inspired about creating experiences together that are not only sensual and pleasurable, but also meaningful and even transformative. We're also optimistic that you'll discover opportunities for intimacy, healing, and growth in the challenges that life will eventually present you with.

You'd probably agree that without the personal anecdotes of how other people have applied the suggestions in these pages to their own situations, this book wouldn't be nearly as helpful. In fact, that's why our clients, acquaintances, and readers of our other books have been so willing to share their stories with you. For them, as for us, it's genuinely rewarding to know that others will benefit from the ideas and insights arising out of one's own real-life experiences.

We all have our own interests, histories, desires, and struggles, and every relationship is unique—which means everyone's perspective is valuable. What you have to say could spark someone else's imagination or help them to better understand their partner or themselves. It could help bring another couple into a closer, deeper, or sexier place together.

So, we'd love to hear from you!

Is there an intimate adventure you've dreamed up? A creative approach to an insecurity or intimacy issue that you've had success with? Or a fun erotic discovery you've made together? You have our undivided attention!

The more possibilities we hear about, the more we can help others to continue evolving and enjoying their own relationships. So this is our invitation to you to keep the conversation going—along with the adventures, the discoveries, the laughter, and, most of all, the love.

With ours,
Mali & Joe
maliandjoe@maliandjoe.com

SEXY DATE IDEAS

When you want inspiration for your next sexy time together, this is a great place to start. You can have endless fun with all of these creative ideas for increasing your intimacy and keeping your sexual connection engaged and energized.

You'll find suggestions throughout this book for how to choose just the right intimate adventure for the two of you, including tips for making it a success and supporting each other when needed, such as when fears or doubts come up. In addition, the pages listed below offer additional information and inspiration.

SEXY CONVERSATION STARTERS

Let's start with some provocative questions that will jumpstart an intimate conversation. Take a question or two along with you on a walk or out to dinner. A little verbal foreplay will open up new avenues for intimacy, deepening your emotional connection and keeping you erotically charged up.

- Check out the Intimacy Inquiry on pages 5–10, the topics on pages 21–22, and the intimate conversation starters on pages

217–222. Remember, even a conversation about *why* a particular topic makes one or both of you nervous can be very connecting.
- Talk about your feelings around nudity. (page 200)
- Have a conversation about a new adventure the two of you are considering trying. (page 18)
- Try out one of the seductive suggestions on pages 201–202.
- Take turns sharing what you each find sexy to hear the other say. (page 203)
- Describe some of the fantasies and desires you had when you were younger—as well as any ways in which those erotic ideas are reflected in who you are today. (page 53)
- Talk about some of the sexual interests and fantasies that *other* people have. (pages 51–52)
- Share some of *your* sexual desires and fantasies. But first, review the guidelines in "Sharing Your Sexual Interests" on pages 53–57.

FOR A SEXY DATE NIGHT OUT

Following are a variety of ideas for an evening out—or, when you have the opportunity, an entire weekend.

- First, before your date, take a few moments to think back to and reconnect with that sense of anticipation you had earlier on in your relationship. You could even cultivate desire for your partner by looking at a photo or two that you love. (pages 60–61)
- Go beyond "dinner and a movie" by experimenting with activities that are new to you both. Exciting new experiences will flood you with adrenaline, the same hormone that was activated when you felt those first rushes of sexual attraction. (pages 193–194)
- Romantically reminisce! Re-create that long hug in the moonlight, or hold hands at that little café you've never forgotten.

- Take your lover on a treasure hunt for the shirt, dress, or sleepwear that looks the sexiest on them. (page 201)
- When you're somewhere that's a good place for people-watching, play "Who Would You Do?" (page 177)
- Pretend that you're single again—together! This intriguing exercise can help you tap back into that feeling of chemistry or sexual energy between you. (pages 173–174)
- Visit a lingerie or sensuality store and check out the sexy accessories, like stockings, stick-on tattoos, body paint, and jewelry. (page 201)
- Attend a sensual art exhibit or performance. (page 194)
- Take a walk by the light of the moon.
- Get a little playful with PDAs, or public displays of affection. (page 203)
- Indulge in a massage for two or a foot reflexology session.
- Play on the "just enough jealousy" edge. After you've read chapter 6, "Jealousy: Another Opportunity for Intimacy (Really!)," talk about what would tease out just a touch of jealousy in each of you. (page 171) Experiment with creating just enough jealousy. (pages 172–173) Walk into a club or party separately and observe each other interact. Or walk through a market or down a city street a little ways apart. (pages 173–175)
- Watch each other flirt. (pages 213–214)
- Take a shibari (a Japanese style of rope bondage) class together. (page 227)
- Go to a kink or BDSM shop or event. (page 227)
- Attend an intimacy event or wild workshop. (pages 215–216)
- Go out on a date with each of you taking on a new identity. (page 194)
- Visit an adult toy store with a positive vibe—or an online pleasure shop—and add to your toy collection. (pages 195–196)

- Visit a communal bathhouse or spa, such as those in Japan, Korea, or Europe, or a clothing-optional hot springs, like those across the U.S., and take the opportunity to become more comfortable in your birthday suits. (pages 200–201)

SEXY DINNER DATE ACTIVITIES

When you're out to dinner together, consider making all non-tantalizing topics off-limits: no work talk and no complaining. Instead, take along a couple of the sexy conversation starters above—or try one of these ideas:

- Reminisce about a sexy adventure you've already had together. You might even make plans to return to the scene of the pleasure when you have the opportunity.
- Talk about a risqué experience you've been planning.
- Play the watcher-watchee game. (pages 174–175)
- Describe what you're going to do to each other later in the evening.
- Plan your next sex vacation. Even if you can only get away for a single night, make plans for a time when you can leave behind your roles as spouses, parents, and wage earners and come back together as lovers. (page 206)
- Mark a map with all the locations you've had a sexy time together. (page 201)
- Tell each other stories about previous sexual experiences you've had. If you're game to try this, be sure to review the guidelines on pages 230–233.

FOR A SEXY DATE NIGHT AT HOME

You'll likely be spending most of your sexy time in your own bedroom, so make it interesting!

- Spend some time in your bedroom creating an ambiance for intimacy. (page 195)
- Romantically reminisce: Play songs you listened to when you first fell in love. Reread notes you wrote to each other early on. Or look through photos of special times you've shared together. (page 62)
- Watch a sophisticated, sexually explicit TV series or an empowering documentary that explores an issue that affects one or both of you personally. Or check out some educational sites that feature instructional videos on everything from sexual communication to self-pleasuring to oral sex techniques. (page 194)
- Turn the lights down and dance naked together. (pages 200–201)
- Walk around your home in search of "pervertibles"—everyday objects that can be used for sensual play, like spatulas, bandanas, neckties, textured bath gloves, feathers, and clothespins. And then, of course, try them out on each other! (page 196)
- Feed each other with your fingers.
- If you have access to a large bathtub or hot tub, float your lover in your arms while they completely relax. (page 200)
- Buy a massager or two—like those shaped for the neck or for kneading out knots in the back—and use them on each other.
- Put into words whatever hot thoughts you're thinking: "It turns me on to see you in those tight jeans!" "I know exactly how you like this." "Watching you take your shirt off makes me want you!" (pages 202–203)
- Dance seductively for your lover while they relax back and admire you. (page 204)
- Read some sexy stories to each other (try searching "erotic fiction").
- Give your lover a sexy striptease or lap dance. (pages 204–205)

- Experiment with other people's turn-ons. (page 204)
- Take some time to explore anal play. (page 208)
- Enjoy some erotica together. (page 213)
- Orally pleasure your partner playing whatever music they would like to be pleasured to.
- Treat your lover to a session of hand sex, or stimulation using only the hands. (pages 206–208)
- Indulge in some sensory awareness practices together, appreciating your bodies as sensual, erotic instruments. (pages 40–42, 45–46)
- Read "A Field Guide of Mindful Lovemaking" together (pages 92–94) and try some of the ideas for bringing more mindfulness into your bedroom.
- Before making love, take a few moments to engage in a ritual that encourages emotional connection. (page 61)
- Experiment with breath and sound practices, like those taught in tantra. (pages 211–212)
- Make love to a variety of music, from the romantic rhythms and passionate melodies of a Spanish guitar, to the soulful vibrations of the cello, to a hypnotic hip-hop jam. (pages 197–198)
- Experiment with ideas for tapping into a feeling of spiritual connection between you. (pages 63–64)
- Make love to yourselves in front of each other—being the witness to each other's self-pleasure. Or self-pleasure, together. (pages 196 and 209)
- If your partner is usually the initiator in the bedroom, try taking the lead—especially if your partner would enjoy it. (page 228)
- Give each other a secret sex name.
- If your lover has a vagina and is willing, take your time exploring the sensitivities and pleasure points of the various areas, including the zone of increased sensitivity typically referred to as the G-spot. (pages 207–208)
- Anytime is a good time to ask, "How is this for you? What can I do to make it even better?"

INTIMATE ADVENTURES AND EROTIC EXPLORATIONS

Finally, here are a few more elaborate ideas for when you have an entire evening or weekend, at home or away.

- Bathe or shower naked together. Or take a shower or hot tub—while blindfolded!
- Gift your lover with an evening at their own personal "sex spa." (page 47)
- Attend an online intimacy or tantra workshop.
- Have your lover painted and photographed by a professional body painter.
- Put on a pussyfest (or a breastfest, assfest, cockfest)—get creative! (pages 65–66)
- Play with a little voyeurism and exhibitionism together. (page 51)
- Try on other people' interests—like knismophilia, pictophilia, and xylophilia. (pages 52–53)
- Give your lover the gift of an ass-worshipping session. (page 52)
- Treat each other to a full-on sensual massage. (pages 198–200)
- Orally pleasure each other at the same time ("69") while focusing all your attention on your senses. (pages 45–46)
- Hold a wet t-shirt contest for one—or for you both!
- Create a silicone replica of you or your partner's private parts. You can pick up a kit online or in a sensuality shop.
- Make love to the passage of time by exploring photos of yourselves when you were younger. Read more about this unusual date night idea on page 134.
- Design an erotic healing experience. Chapter 4, "The Psychology of Phenomenal Sex" (pages 69–94), is filled with ideas for helping your lover make new, positive, and pleasurable associations with something that makes them feel anxious or insecure. The many examples will inspire you to think creatively about

what might assist your lover in opening up to more love and pleasure.

- Take some sexy selfies to capture the sensuality, passion, and intimacy between you. (page 211)
- Stir up some sexual creativity through fantasy play. If the idea makes you nervous, check out the suggestions on pages 48–49.
- Explore a variety of creative approaches to oral sex. See the ideas on pages 47 and 209–210.
- Pleasure your partner while they enjoy a rendezvous with an imaginary lover. (pages 216–217)
- Explore fantasies that are entirely beyond the realm of possibility. (page 53)
- Share some of your fantasies with each other. First, be sure you both read the section "Sharing Your Sexual Interests" for ideas on how to do this successfully. (pages 53–57)
- Indulge your partner's fantasy by playing out their sexy scenario with them. (pages 216–217)
- Play with the power of eroticism. Chapter 5, "The Healing Power of Eroticism" (pages 95–136), offers an abundance of ways to help a partner let go of limiting beliefs, quiet their self-critical voice, overcome perceived limitations, and heal from their past. By making something erotic, or "arousing sexual desire," you can help free your lover from something that's been preventing them from experiencing love, connection, intimacy, and pleasure.
- Sensuously touch your lover while they relax in front of a mirror and take in their own image as an erotic art form. (page 205)
- Have sex or orgasm with your eyes open or while looking into each other's eyes. (pages 61–62)

IN GRATITUDE

We are beyond grateful to the many generous and loving people who have encouraged, educated, and inspired us to be as sensitive, as inclusive, and as real as possible.

Yolanda D'Aquino, our oh-so-brilliant editor, for your wisdom, compassion, and insight, which grace every page. Visiting that vulva wall with you is at the top of our "intimate adventures" bucket list!

Sarah Dunn, for being infinitely positive and supportive of all our endeavors. And Lana Apple, for never allowing us to take ourselves too seriously. You are the perfect daughters for us!

Isabel Mize, for your truly unconditional love and your unshakable personal and professional belief in the value of our message.

Gerise Pappas, for encouraging us to lead with our love story.

Laura Marshall, for your sage and gentle guidance all the way through. And Tom Towey III, for your unwavering faith in love.

Rachel Noyes, for your unique perspectives and abundant enthusiasm for this project.

Marybeth Giefer, for always reminding us that life is a love adventure.

Lisa Vincent, for your thoughtfulness, your attentiveness—and your persistence!

Lilou Mace, for admonishing Mali not to be a good girl.

Janet Brown and Kayla Dunnigan, for your spot-on sensitivity.

Meghan Dunn, Tim Taylor, Maile Reilly, and Doug Hanford, for all the enlightening conversations.

John Hatem, for the lesson in the art of seduction.

Rick Schaffer, for materializing at just the right moment.

And finally, for all manner of cheerleading, hand-holding, inspiration, reflections, suggestions, and expertise, our heartfelt thanks to Rod Bacon, Fran Bennett, Paul Beyers, Sandi Bowen, Michael DeSario, Deanna Dudney, Anna Embree, Carmen Gamper, Paul Francis Giefer, France-Laude Gohard, Michael Grossman, Gina Inez, Jeromy Johnson, Jonathan Kovac, Anna Kyshynska, Reeshemah Langham, Kelly LaValley, Aimee McCabe, Kristi McCullough, Abby Minot, Megan Monique, Rod Morgan, Ellie Oldroyd, Karlyn Pipes, Brian Scherer, and Joanne Sprott.

About Mali & Joe

Like many other couples in a new relationship, we experienced a deeply profound, almost magical feeling of connection when we began dating almost two decades ago. Not wanting this experience to end, we began an exploration into love, intimacy, and sex—and especially the question of how two people could keep their connection passionate, loving, and alive indefinitely.

As we dedicated ourselves to this question, we began to coach singles and couples in applying our discoveries to transform their own lives and relationships. And as we witnessed the people we coached become more accepting toward themselves and more connected to those they loved, we decided to put all our ideas, tools, and techniques into a book so more people could have access to them. That's how *The Soulmate Experience: A Practical Guide to Creating Extraordinary Relationships* was born. Five years later, we followed that up with *The Soulmate Lover: A Guide to Passionate and Lasting Love, Sex, and Intimacy*.

We've been thrilled by how many people our books have touched over the years. Every time someone tells us how one of our ideas has positively transformed them or their relationship—or saved it altogether—we know we made the right choice to spend the years it took us to write these books.

Intimate relationships are special in that they give us the opportunity to explore deep, erotic connection with another human being. And yet sexuality—which is so often tangled up with insecurity, jealousy, inhibition, shame, and self-consciousness—can be quite challenging for couples. Helping people successfully work with the many kinds of sexual challenges that can arise in a relationship helped us make the decision to, once again, share our ideas and our clients' success stories in this book, *Wild Monogamy*.

We spend a lot of time together: we live together, we write together, and we coach together. And after almost two decades, we're still exploring love, sex, and relationships. We're still falling in love, we're still making love, and our sexual connection is as strong as ever. And we're confident that the ideas we share in our books will help you experience more love, more intimacy, and more connection in your life.

In love,
Mali & Joe

RESOURCES

To keep our relationships feeling alive and filled with potential, it helps to have sources of new ideas and perspectives. So here are a few of our personal favorites, listed alphabetically by author. Check out our website, MaliAndJoe.com, for up-to-date podcast recommendations.

For Each Other: Sharing Sexual Intimacy. First published in 1982, this classic by brilliant therapist Lonnie Barbach is still amazingly relevant today.

The Gifts of Imperfection: Let Go of Who You Think You're Supposed to Be and Embrace Who You Are. A beautiful book by researcher Brené Brown that will help you recognize and let go of shame and striving for perfection and know that you are worthy of love and belonging.

Curvy Girl Sex: 101 Body-Positive Positions to Empower Your Sex Life. In addition to recommending specific positions, sex educator Elle Chase helps people of all shapes and sizes feel sexy, self-confident, and desirable.

Great Sex Starts at 50: Age-Proof Your Libido and Transform Your Sex Life. Honest, straightforward, and encouraging with a good dose of humor, this book by sex expert Tracey Cox will have you feeling more confident with your sexuality no matter your age. She offers sensible and creative approaches to all the usual issues that come with aging, including lots of advice for talking about it all with your partner.

The Vagina Bible: The Vulva and the Vagina—Separating the Myth from the Medicine. Worthy of its title, this comprehensive and straightforward guide from OB-GYN Jen Gunter covers practically every question one might have about the vulva and vagina.

Because It Feels Good: A Woman's Guide to Sexual Pleasure and Satisfaction. Sexual health educator and researcher Debby Herbenick empowers women with information and guidance to create satisfying, fun, intimate, and pleasurable sex lives.

She Comes First: The Thinking Man's Guide to Pleasuring a Woman. The classic by sex therapist Ian Kerner. If you're reading along and begin to feel it's taking too long to get warmed up, don't give up: skip to the second half of the book for Kerner's detailed guide to cunnilingus.

Sexual Intelligence: What We Really Want from Sex and How to Get It. Sex therapist Marty Klein offers a new vision of how to discover what we've really been desiring from sex and open ourselves up to experiencing that, including addressing issues with desire in long-term relationships.

Magnificent Sex: Lessons from Extraordinary Lovers. Sex therapist Peggy J. Kleinplatz and clinical psychologist A. Dana Ménard present the fascinating and insightful results of their extensive interviews and research into the lives of people who are having extraordinary sex.

Tell Me What You Want: The Science of Sexual Desire and How It Can Help You Improve Your Sex Life. Written in the clear, warm tone that characterizes all of researcher Justin J. Lehmiller's work, this book will help you feel more comfortable with your own erotic imagination and offers guidance for talking about your desires with your partner.

Attached: The New Science of Adult Attachment and How It Can Help You Find—and Keep—Love. A classic work on attachment theory by psychiatrist Amir Levine and psychologist Rachel S. F. Heller that helps you identify and understand your attachment style, and that of your partner or prospective partner, to help you build stronger, more fulfilling connections.

Partners in Passion: A Guide to Great Sex, Emotional Intimacy and Long-Term Love. Married couple and neo-tantra teachers Mark A. Michaels and Patricia Johnson bring their knowledge and perspective to every aspect of long-term relating, from building sexual trust to adventuring together. Thoroughly researched, thoughtfully written, and packed with useful exercises.

The Erotic Mind: Unlocking the Inner Sources of Passion and Fulfillment. This classic by psychologist and sexologist Jack Morin is filled with insights. Eroticism, Morin says, is "the process through which sex becomes meaningful." He talks about the idea that remaining attracted to a long-term partner is a choice. "The ability to sustain attraction is, to a significant degree, a conscious decision, an act of will," he says. "It is your responsibility to be actively receptive, to open your eyes enthusiastically to the beauty of your lover."

Come as You Are: The Surprising New Science That Will Transform Your Sex Life. The 2021 revised edition updates and improves on sex educator Emily Nagoski's bestseller on the science behind arousal, desire, and pleasure.

The Ultimate Guide to Seduction and Foreplay: Techniques and Strategies for Mind-Blowing Sex. This gem by sexologists Jessica O'Reilly and Marla Renee Stewart contains plenty of excellent suggestions for talking about sex—including insightful questions and examples of sexy talk—as well as lots of fun techniques to experiment with. We especially appreciate their chapter on eroticizing daily interactions as a "seduction strategy" for busy people.

Better Than I Ever Expected: Straight Talk About Sex After Sixty. Affirming, entertaining, and encouraging, as is everything sex expert Joan Price does. The many quotes and stories from older people about everything from what helps them feel positively about their bodies and sex lives to what helps them get turned on and feel sexy will leave you feeling uplifted and ready to age up.

Naked at Our Age: Talking Out Loud About Senior Sex. Joan Price brings a host of experts in the fields of relationships and sexuality together to address age-related challenges and joys as expressed in the many candid stories from everyday people.

Peak Sexual Experience: Techniques for Better Sex, Better Loving, and Greater Intimacy in Your Relationship. Prolific psychologist John Selby's classic in the field, with lots of ideas to ponder if you're interested in exploring the depths of the transcendent feelings of connection possible through a sexual relationship, especially with a long-term partner.

NOTES

2 Six Keys to Erotic Adventures

1. David Schnarch, *Passionate Marriage: Keeping Love and Intimacy Alive in Committed Relationships* (New York: W. W. Norton, 2009).
2. In *Tell Me What You Want: The Science of Sexual Desire and How It Can Help You Improve Your Sex Life* (New York: Hachette Books, 2018), social psychologist Justin J. Lehmiller discusses at length the fact that people's fantasies have diverse origins, including demographic factors, personality traits, and their sexual and relationship histories and experiences.
3. Even if someone is disturbed by the content of their sexual imagination and it creates a lot of guilt and shame for them, it can be quite challenging or impossible to eradicate the fantasy completely. If the person is motivated, however, and perhaps with the help of a counselor or therapist, they could potentially modify their fantasy, or learn to fantasize about something else, in a way that still taps into what turns them on but isn't as troubling for them. (Justin J. Lehmiller, interview with Dan Savage, *Savage Lovecast* podcast episode 626, Oct. 23, 2018.) In *The Erotic Mind: Unlocking the Inner Sources of Sexual Passion and Fulfillment* (New York: HarperCollins, 1995), legendary sex therapist Jack Morin offers a seven-step process for modifying a troublesome turn-on. Finally, for fantasies that have their origins in some kind of trauma, it's possible that working with those fantasies, rather than trying to eradicate them, can actually be therapeutic and a way of healing from that trauma (Ian Kerner, interview with Justin Lehmiller, *Sex & Psychology* podcast episode 29, April 9, 2021).

3 Erotic Versatility

1. Numerous studies have demonstrated links between sexual activity and orgasms and such health benefits as the following:
   • Lowering the incidence of prostate cancer: Jennifer R. Rider et al., "Ejaculation Frequency and Risk of Prostate Cancer: Updated Results with an Additional Decade of Follow-up," *European Urology* 70(6), 2016: 974–82. DOI: 10.1016/j.eururo.2016.03.027
   • Strengthening the pelvic floor muscles: Dulcegleika Vilas Boas Sartori et al., "Pelvic Floor Muscle Strength Is Correlated with Sexual Function," *Investigative and Clinical Urology* 62(1), 2021: 79–84. DOI:10.4111/icu.20190248
   • Reducing heart disease: Susan A. Hall et al., "Sexual Activity, Erectile Dysfunction, and Incident Cardiovascular Events," *The American Journal of Cardiology* 105(2), 2010: 192–97. DOI:10.1016/j.amjcard.2009.08.671
   • Living longer: George Davey Smith, Stephen Frankel, and John Yarnell, "Sex and Death: Are They Related? Findings from the Caerphilly Cohort Study," *BMJ* 315(7123), 1997: 1641–44. DOI: 10.1136/bmj.315.7123.1641
2. See, for example, Jessica R. Wood et al., "Was It Good for You Too?: An Analysis of Gender Differences in Oral Sex Practices and Pleasure Ratings Among Heterosexual Canadian University Students," *The Canadian Journal of Human Sexuality* 25(1), 2016: 21–29. DOI: 10.3138/cjhs.251-A2. And Sarah N. Bell., "What Happens in a Hook Up?: Young Women's Behaviors, Emotions, and Pleasures," Dissertation, Univ. of Michigan, 2018. ORCID iD: 0000-0002-8796-7892
3. Schnarch, *Passionate Marriage*.
4. Chrisanna Northrup, Pepper Schwartz, and James Witte, *The Normal Bar: The Surprising Secrets of Happy Couples and What They Reveal About Creating a New Normal in Your Relationship* (New York: Harmony Books, 2014).
5. In Justin J. Lehmiller's large survey of Americans, as described in *Tell Me What You Want,* 97% of respondents reported having sexual fantasies. In *The Erotic Mind,* Jack Morin suggests that people who say they rarely or never fantasize are similar to people who say they never dream: they just don't pay close enough attention to their arousing thoughts. Rather than detailed fantasies, they might experience fragments or fleeting thoughts or images of an erotic nature. These "unrecognized fantasies," as Morin calls them, are created by the mind and are part of one's erotic imagination and thus "fantasy" life.
6. Jesse Bering, *Perv: The Sexual Deviant in All of Us* (New York: Scientific American, 2013).

7. There may be some interests it would be wise to keep private indefinitely, such as those involving children, animals, or anything dangerous or illegal. This is a complex issue. For example, consider someone being tormented by fantasies involving minors—someone who has never acted on such thoughts and never wants to, but is greatly troubled by them and wants help reducing or eliminating them. In some locations (such as the U.S.), reporting requirements, or a therapist's interpretation of those requirements, might mean that if this person sought professional help, they could end up being reported to authorities. For this reason, someone who is facing this difficult dilemma might want to research other resources, including anonymous online support groups. When it comes to the question of whether to share such thoughts or desires with a partner, weigh what you know about your partner with the possibility that fears or judgments could get triggered. Whether or not you already feel shame and guilt around your interests, having shame layered on you by someone you love, even if that's not their intention, could make things more difficult. On the other hand, imagine how healing, and bonding, it might be when someone is able to share their "deep dark secret" with their partner and receives compassion for their struggle and support in finding help. As we said, this is complicated—not only for people with such interests, but potentially their partners and even their therapists.
8. Justin J. Lehmiller, interview with April Lampert and Amy Baldwin, *Shameless Sex* podcast episode 98, March 19, 2019.
9. Amy Muise et al., "Keeping the Spark Alive: Being Motivated to Meet a Partner's Sexual Needs Sustains Sexual Desire in Long-Term Romantic Relationships," *Social Psychological and Personality Science* 4(3), 2012: 267–73. DOI: 10.1177/1948550612457185
10. See David J. Ley, *Insatiable Wives: Women Who Stray and the Men Who Love Them* (Lanham, MD: Rowman and Littlefield, 2009).
11. Marty Klein, *Sexual Intelligence: What We Really Want from Sex—and How to Get It* (New York: HarperCollins, 2012).
12. From Lisa Wade, *American Hookup: The New Culture of Sex on Campus* (New York: W. W. Norton, 2017). Wade, a sociologist, says the majority of students in her research "would prefer more meaningful connections with others."
13. Morin, *The Erotic Mind*.
14. In *Not Always in the Mood: The New Science of Men, Sex, and Relationships* (Lanham, MD: Rowman and Littlefield, 2019), Sarah Hunter Murray says that "communication and romantic settings [are] factors that facilitate men's

sexual interest. And the thing that ties these two pieces together is that they both facilitate the experiences of closeness and intimate, emotional connection." She continues: "In fact, emotional closeness is so important to men's experience of sexual desire that if you're *not* feeling emotionally close, chances are his desire won't be there."

15. David Schnarch, "Joy with Your Underwear Down," *Psychology Today*, June 9, 2016. www.psychologytoday.com/us/articles/196912/joy-your-underwear-down
16. John Selby, *Peak Sexual Experience: Techniques for Better Sex, Better Loving, and Greater Intimacy in Your Relationship* (New York: Warner Books, 1992).
17. Selby, *Peak Sexual Experience:*

4 The Psychology of Phenomenal Sex

1. This concept, in which two people help sculpt each other into their best selves, has been termed the Michelangelo effect.
2. See, for example, Martin E. P. Seligman, *Learned Optimism: How to Change Your Mind and Your Life* (New York: Vintage Books, 2006).
3. Lori A. Brotto, *Better Sex through Mindfulness: How Women Can Cultivate Desire* (Vancouver: Greystone Books, 2018).
4. These touching practices, in which arousal and orgasms are not the goal, are similar to the sensate focus exercises developed by sex researchers Masters and Johnson in the 1960s to help people learn how to enjoy the simple pleasures of touching.

5 The Healing Power of Eroticism

1. Morin, *The Erotic Mind.*
2. This review of many studies found an average length of 5.1 to 5.5 in. (13 to 14 cm). Bruce M. King, "Average-Size Erect Penis: Fiction, Fact, and the Need for Counseling," *Journal of Sex & Marital Therapy* 47:1, 2021: 80–89. DOI: 10.1080/0092623X.2020.1787279
3. Brené Brown, *The Gifts of Imperfection: Let Go of Who You Think You're Supposed to Be and Embrace Who You Are* (Culver City, MN: Hazelden, 2010).
4. In *Tell Me What You Want,* Lehmiller reports that in his research "victims of sex crimes were more likely than nonvictims to fantasize about almost all aspects of BDSM (dominance being the primary exception)" and argues that "these fantasies are adaptive coping mechanisms for dealing with previous sexual trauma and, if anything, should be viewed as a sign of psychological resilience."

5. Estimates vary widely on the prevalence of erectile dysfunction. Although rates increase with age, ED affects younger men as well.
6. Other techniques for gaining more ejaculatory control or lasting longer during penetrative sex include momentarily moving the attention to something nonsexual, slowing down until the arousal level lessens, and squeezing the tip of the penis until the intensity of the sensations subsides.
7. This statistic comes from a comprehensive review of studies published in Elisabeth A. Lloyd, *The Case of the Female Orgasm: Bias in the Science of Evolution* (Cambridge, MA: Harvard University Press, 2006). In addition, about 50% of heterosexual women sometimes orgasm through intercourse alone, 20% never orgasm through intercourse, and 5% never orgasm at all.
8. Ogi Ogas and Sai Gaddam, *A Billion Wicked Thoughts: What the Internet Tells Us About Sexual Relationships* (New York: Plume, 2011).
9. Morin, *The Erotic Mind*.

6 Jealousy

1. Northrup et al., *The Normal Bar.*

7 Playing in the Garden of Eden

1. David A. Frederick et al., "What Keeps Passion Alive? Sexual Satisfaction Is Associated with Sexual Communication, Mood Setting, Sexual Variety, Oral Sex, Orgasm, and Sex Frequency in a National U.S. Study," *Journal of Sex Research* 54(2), 2017: 186–201. DOI: 10.1080/00224499.2015.1137854. Jennifer L. Montesi et al., "The Specific Importance of Communicating About Sex to Couples' Sexual and Overall Relationship Satisfaction," *Journal of Social and Personal Relationships* 28(5): 2011, 591–609. DOI:10.1177/0265407510386833. Julia R. Heiman et al., "Sexual Satisfaction and Relationship Happiness in Midlife and Older Couples in Five Countries," *Archives of Sexual Behavior* 40(4): 2011, 741–53. DOI: 10.1007/s10508-010-9703-3. Amy Muise, Elaine Giang, and Emily A. Impett, "Post Sex Affectionate Exchanges Promote Sexual and Relationship Satisfaction," *Archives of Sexual Behavior* 43(7): 2014, 1391–1402. DOI: 10.1007/s10508-014-0305-3. Chris Rissel et al., "Heterosexual Experience and Recent Heterosexual Encounters Among Australian Adults: The Second Australian Study of Health and Relationships," *Sexual Health* 11(5): 2014, 416–26. DOI: 10.1071/SH14105
2. Frederick et al., "What Keeps Passion Alive?"

3. Many studies verify these facts. Also see Christopher Ryan and Cacilda Jethá, *Sex at Dawn: How We Mate, Why We Stray, and What It Means for Modern Relationships* (New York: Harper Perennial, 2011).
4. See Debby Herbenick and Vanessa Schick, *Read My Lips: A Complete Guide to the Vagina and Vulva* (London: Rowman & Littlefield, 2011).
5. Andrew J. Sun and Michael L. Eisenberg, "Association Between Marijuana Use and Sexual Frequency in the United States: A Population-Based Study," *The Journal of Sexual Medicine* 14(11), 2017: 1342–47. DOI: 10.1016/j.jsxm.2017.09.005. Becky K. Lynn et al., "The Relationship Between Marijuana Use Prior to Sex and Sexual Function in Women," *Sexual Medicine* 7(2), 2019: 192–97. DOI: 10.1016/j.esxm.2019.01.003

8 Monogamy with Benefits

1. Frederick et al., "What Keeps Passion Alive?" In addition, this study of 2,021 adults found that 18% of men and 10% of women had engaged in a threesome: Herbenick et al., "Sexual Diversity in the United States: Results from a Nationally Representative Probability Sample of Adult Women and Men," *PLOS ONE* 12(7), 2017. DOI: 10.1371/journal.pone.0181198
2. Estimates vary, but between 2% and 5% of the U.S. adult population currently practice some type of consensual nonmonogamy, and around 20% have tried it at some point. Several studies show these numbers to be higher in queer relationships.

INDEX